Field Guide
to the Chest X-Ray

Anthony McCluffy

D1516194

Field Guide to the Chest X-Ray

Wallace T. Miller, MD
Professor of Radiology
University of Pennsylvania
Philadelphia, PA

Wallace T. Miller, Jr., MD
Assistant Professor of Radiology
University of Pennsylvania
Philadelphia, PA

LIPPINCOTT WILLIAMS & WILKINS
A **Wolters Kluwer** Company
Philadelphia · Baltimore · New York · London
Buenos Aires · Hong Kong · Sydney · Tokyo

Editor: Richard Winters
Developmental Editor: Sara Lauber
Marketing Manager: Kathleen Neely
Project Editor: Ulita Lushnycky
Design Coordinator: Mario Fernandez

351 West Camden Street
Baltimore, Maryland 21201-2436 USA

227 East Washington Square
Philadelphia, PA 19106

Printed in the United States of America

First Edition, 1999

Library of Congress Cataloging-in-Publication Data

Miller, Wallace T.
    Field guide to the chest X-ray /   Wallace T. Miller, Wallace T.
Miller, Jr. — 1st ed.
        p. cm.
    ISBN 0-7817-2028-1
    1. Chest—Radiography.   2. Chest Radiography—Atlases.
3. Diagnosis, Differential.   4. Chest—Diseases—Diagnosis.
I. Miller, Wallace T., 1958–   .   II. Title.
    [DNLM: 1. Lung Diseases—diagnosis.   2. Lung—radiography.   WF
600   M6518f   1999]
RC941.M546   1999
617.5′407572—dc21
DNLM/DLC   99-17626
for Library of Congress   CIP

To purchase additional copies of this book, call our customer service department at **(800) 638-3030** or fax orders to **(301) 824-7390**. International customers should call **(301) 714-2324**.

                                                00 01 02 03
                                             2 3 4 5 6 7 8 9 10

Preface

In the chest, the plain film remains the major tool in the identification and exclusion of chest diseases. Understanding the findings on the routine chest film increases our understanding of a patient's disease and often obviates the necessity for more complex diagnostic tests.

The cardinal tenent of chest radiology is: structures are identifiable because they contain air or are outlined or surrounded by air. The lungs are filled with air and various pulmonary diseases cause alterations in the lung patterns which are easily recognizable and give us accurate insight into the patient's disease. In addition, the lungs are often affected by systemic disease; the changes created may allow us to recognize a particular systemic disease, even though the lungs are only minimally involved.

Most of the other structures in the chest are visible because they are adjacent to, or surrounded by, the air in the lung. Thus the diaphragm, chest wall, heart, aorta, and other mediastinal structures are visible because they are adjacent to the air containing lung. Abnormalities of these structures may be recognized because of their altered contour as they project into the lungs.

Other structures which normally are relatively invisible may become visible when diseased. The parietal and visceral pleura are normally so thin as to be basically invisible, but when a pleural mass or pleural effusion develops in the pleural space, these structures become visible by displacing the air containing lung. Likewise, a chest wall mass may become visible if it projects into the chest cavity and encroaches on the lungs.

In addition to the air containing lungs and structures outlined by them, the other important radiographic structure in the chest on the plain film is the bony skeleton. The vertebral bodies and the ribs may be altered by intrinsic disease or by adjacent processes that involve the bones. These alterations may allow one to recognize localized or systemic bony disease.

This text will deal with radiographic patterns that occur in the chest and which are recognizable to the interested observer.

Unfortunately, there are few things in medicine that create a pattern so specific that a single definitive diagnosis can be made. In most instances, there are a number of entities which create a certain pattern. Our job is to recognize the radiographic pattern and to arrive at a differential diagnosis of that particular pattern.

Pattern recognition is actually the easy part. Most of us can learn to recognize the various patterns which occur in the lungs or surrounding structures. The hard part is to take this information, along with the clinical history, and to narrow the myriad of differential possibilities into several or perhaps a single entity. This is the art of radiology, and something which any physician can learn with practice.

On the following pages, a list of differential diagnoses will be suggested for each radiographic pattern. These lists are not all inclusive, but do include the major diseases which create a certain radiographic pattern. Some attempt will be made to suggest clinical or radiographic parameters that may narrow the differential.

Contents

1 Diffuse Lung Disease

The first pattern on a chest film to discuss is diffuse disease. Though the entire lung often is involved by a diffuse process, lung disease still may be considered to be diffuse if only part of the lung is involved. Both lungs, however, must be involved in a relatively symmetrical fashion.

ALVEOLAR DISEASE

Only three areas of the lung can be involved in a diffuse process: the vessels, the alveoli or air spaces, and the supporting structures. Other chapters deal with various vascular patterns that are indicative of various diseases as well as with hyperinflation or expansion of the air spaces. This chapter deals with various conditions that opacify the air spaces or infiltrate the supporting structures (i.e., the interstitium).

Diffuse alveolar or air-space disease involves filling of the alveolus by some type of fluid (e.g., pus, blood, water). Findings on the chest film that indicate alveolar filling include:

1. The density created in the lung usually has irregular or "fluffy" margins.
2. The density usually is confluent, which is the major hallmark of alveolar disease. As a filling process progresses from one alveolus or acinus to another, the area of involvement becomes solid and dense.
3. The "silhouette sign" occurs. Most of the structures in the thorax are visualized because of air in the lung. Therefore, when the lung becomes opacified, the silhouette of the structures adjacent to the opacified lung, such as the heart, diaphragm, aorta, and chest wall, is lost. This occurrence has been termed the *silhouette sign*.
4. An "air bronchogram" frequently is present. If the bronchi remain filled with air as the air spaces opacify, then these bronchi, which ordinarily are invisible in the aerated lung, now become visible (i.e., an air bronchogram). Both the silhouette sign and the air bronchogram are indicative of an alveolar or air-space process.
5. In some patients, confluence does not occur, but multiple "acinar" nodules with irregular margins that resemble tiny rosettes do. This is most characteristic of diffuse bronchoalveolar carcinoma, but it sometimes occurs in other alveolar diseases as well.
6. Diffuse air-space disease may involve the lung in a very even manner, so that no one part is distinguishable from another. Often, however, air-space disease involves the central more than the peripheral portions of the lung, thereby creating a butterfly or a bat-wing pattern.
7. Alveolar diseases generally are acute diseases and change rapidly over time.

Causes

The causes of diffuse alveolar disease include:

1. Pulmonary edema.
2. Diffuse pulmonary hemorrhage.
3. Diffuse pulmonary infection.
4. Chronic alveolar disease.
    A. Pulmonary alveolar proteinosis.
    B. Diffuse bronchoalveolar carcinoma.

Pulmonary Edema

Cardiac. Alveolar edema is only one manifestation of cardiac failure. Large vessels and interstitial edema are earlier manifestations of heart failure. Cardiac failure in general as well as its various manifestations are discussed in Chapter 12.

Cardiac alveolar edema is the classic example of diffuse air-space or alveolar disease. This is a common manifestation of heart failure and the pattern usually associated with severe heart failure, but pulmonary edema must start as an interstitial process. This is because the blood vessels lie in the interstitium, and interstitial edema must precede alveolar edema. Usually, the transition from interstitial to alveolar edema occurs quite rapidly, and the pattern of interstitial edema is not visualized.

The classic picture of cardiac alveolar edema is central or perihilar consolidation with some sparing of the periphery of the lung fields (see Fig. 12.3). This edema often is symmetrical. It is just as common, however, for cardiac pulmonary edema to be asymmetrical, with one lung being much more involved than the other, or to be "patchy," with multiple patches of alveolar edema that resemble pneumonia or aspiration (Fig. 1.1). For the most part, the uneven distribution of this pulmonary edema cannot be explained. The distribution of edema tends to shift from day to day, so even though it may remain uneven, the areas of consolidation will differ over time. This changing pattern of alveolar consolidation helps to identify cardiac pulmonary edema as a cause of patchy lung opacification.

Cardiac pulmonary edema often is accompanied by cardiomegaly, but the absence of cardiomegaly does not exclude the diagnosis. Patients with an acute

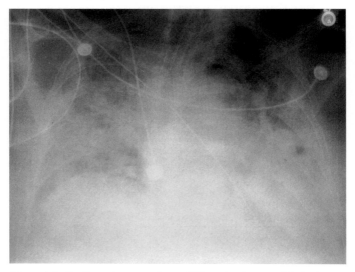

Figure 1.1. Cardiac pulmonary edema. Diffuse alveolar consolidation is present in a rather patchy fashion. This is quite characteristic of cardiac pulmonary edema. (For the classic butterfly or bat-wing pattern, see Fig. 12.3.)

cardiac problem, such as myocardial infarction or an abrupt onset of cardiac arrhythmia, do not have time for the heart to dilate. Therefore, they may have severe pulmonary edema with a normal-size heart.

Radiographic resolution of cardiac pulmonary edema may lag behind clinical resolution of the symptoms of edema. Resolution usually is symmetrical but also may occur in an asymmetrical and unpredictable fashion. Therefore, most of the edema may have resolved completely while one area of lung with fairly extensive pulmonary edema remains.

Noncardiac. Common causes of noncardiac pulmonary edema include:

1. Adult respiratory distress syndrome (ARDS).
2. Drug and transfusion reactions.
3. Smoke inhalation and near-drowning.
4. Fluid overload.
5. Fat embolism.
6. Neurogenic edema.

Though this list is incomplete, it includes most of the major causes of noncardiac pulmonary edema.

Noncardiac pulmonary edema usually cannot be distinguished from cardiac pulmonary edema, and the diagnosis frequently is established on the basis of clinical history. Cardiac size may be of some help in suggesting the correct diagnosis, but the heart may be large in patients noncardiac edema and normal in patients with cardiac edema.

ADULT RESPIRATORY DISTRESS SYNDROME. The most common cause of noncardiac edema in the hospital setting is ARDS. In this condition, alveolar–capillary injury occurs secondary to a variety of causes, such as pulmonary or nonpulmonary infection, shock, trauma, oxygen toxicity, and so on. As a result, fluid leaks from the damaged capillaries into the alveoli, thereby causing diffuse alveolar consolidation (Fig. 1.2*A*). Early in the course of ARDS, this consolidation usually cannot be distinguished from cardiac pulmonary edema and often has a central or perihilar distribution. As ARDS persists, the pulmonary edema becomes more homogeneous and the lung more diffusely and symmetrically involved (Fig. 1.2*B*). At this stage, one usually can distinguish ARDS from cardiac pulmonary edema; however, degrees of cardiac failure or fluid overload can influence the picture of ARDS and make it appear to be either worse or better than it actually is.

The presence of air bronchograms in a patient with pulmonary edema is suggestive of ARDS. This is because well-defined air bronchograms are less common in patients with cardiac pulmonary edema.

Infection in patients with ARDS is almost impossible to recognize, because superimposed pneumonia also has an alveolar distribution and focal infiltrates often are not recognized. Similarly, in patient with ARDS induced by pneumonia or aspiration, the initial infiltrates caused by these processes gradually disappear in 1 or 2 days as the more diffuse picture of ARDS becomes established (Fig. 1.3).

DRUG AND TRANSFUSION REACTIONS. Pulmonary edema may be caused by a hypersensitivity reaction to various drugs. The best-known drugs that cause this type of reaction are morphine and heroin, but almost any drug, including antibiotics, diuretics, nitrofurantoin, interleukin-2, and so on, can sometimes

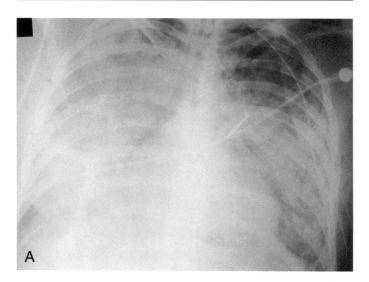

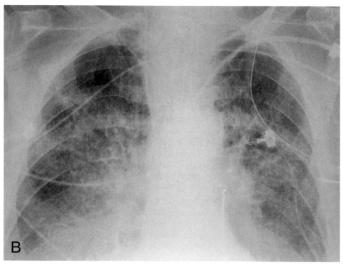

Figure 1.2. Adult respiratory distress syndrome. **A.** Pulmonary edema is somewhat more marked on the right than on the left. Note the air bronchograms in both lungs and loss of the right heart border. **B.** A later stage of disease in another patient. The syndrome now is very diffuse and somewhat homogeneous.

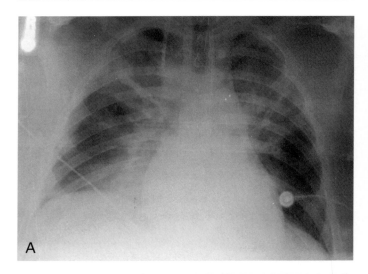

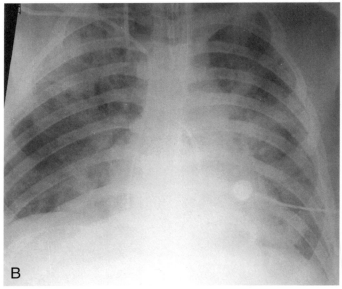

Figure 1.3. Adult respiratory distress syndrome secondary to aspiration. **A.** Patchy aspiration. **B.** Diffuse ARDS masking the previous aspiration pneumonia 2 days later.

cause this reaction. Blood transfusions are a common cause of allergic pulmonary edema, but like many hypersensitivity reactions, the edema usually disappears in 24 to 48 hours if the patient is not re-exposed.

SMOKE INHALATION AND NEAR-DROWNING. Smoke inhalation and near-drowning also are occasional causes of noncardiac pulmonary edema (Fig. 1.4). Fat embolism, which generally is associated with trauma patients, usually with long bone fractures, is another cause of a delayed appearance of ARDS. In all of these entities, patients initially may appear to be quite normal and even have a normal chest film. Several hours to 48 hours later, pulmonary edema usually develops suddenly.

Toxic inhalation of various gases, particularly acids, also can lead to pulmonary edema. Among these gases include those from sulfuric, hydrochloric, and nitric acid. Silo filler's disease creates such an acid as well: nitric acid is formed when N_2O_5 is inhaled and combined with water. In addition, inhalation of a large burden of organic dust may cause noncardiac pulmonary edema in susceptible individuals because of an acute allergic reaction to antigens in the dust.

FLUID OVERLOAD. Pulmonary edema commonly occurs from fluid overload even when the patient's heart is normal. It cannot be distinguished from congestive heart failure.

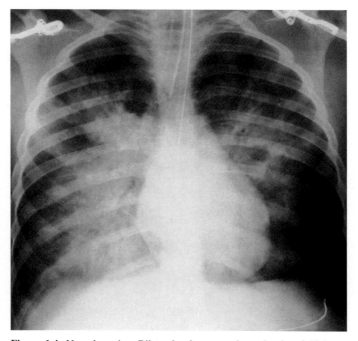

Figure 1.4. Near-drowning. Bilateral pulmonary edema developed 12 hours after this 19-year-old man was removed from the bottom of a pool. The chest film was normal 12 hours earlier.

Diffuse Lung Disease

FAT EMBOLISM. Fat embolism is another cause of noncardiac pulmonary edema. Patients with long bone fractures can develop an ARDS picture from fat emboli.

NEUROGENIC EDEMA. In some patients with neurologic problems involving the posterior fossa, pulmonary edema may occur on a neurogenic basis. Neurogenic pulmonary edema and edema from fat emboli cannot be distinguished from other causes of leaky capillaries (e.g., ARDS).

Diffuse Pulmonary Hemorrhage

Focal pulmonary hemorrhage can be caused by bleeding from several causes, but diffuse pulmonary hemorrhage usually has a systemic cause. Common causes of diffuse pulmonary hemorrhage include:

---

1. Lymphoproliferative malignancy with a bleeding diathesis.
2. Vasculitis, such as Wegener's granulomatosis or systemic lupus erythematosus.
3. Renal disease, such as Goodpasture's syndrome or rapidly progressive glomerulonephritis.
4. Idiopathic pulmonary hemosiderosis.

Like the other diffuse alveolar diseases, diffuse pulmonary hemorrhage usually cannot be distinguished from pulmonary edema. Hemopytsis is variably present or absent in patients with diffuse pulmonary hemorrhage, but anemia is virtually always present. Hemoptysis or acute anemia often is the critical clue suggestive of the diagnosis of pulmonary hemorrhage. Bronchoscopic demonstration of blood-filled airways or hemosiderin-laden macrophages in a biopsy specimen can confirm the suspected diagnosis of pulmonary hemorrhage.

Most diseases that cause pulmonary hemorrhage also may cause other problems that cannot be distinguished on chest films from pulmonary hemorrhage. This often makes the radiographic diagnosis of diffuse hemorrhage difficult to establish. In particular, diffuse infection and pulmonary edema may occur in many diseases that cause pulmonary hemorrhage.

Hematologic Causes.   Diffuse pulmonary hemorrhage probably is seen most commonly in patients with hematologic malignancies who are receiving drug therapy and have very low platelet counts. It also occurs in patients with other bleeding diatheses and in those with disseminated intravascular coagulation. In the later patients, it may be indistinguishable from ARDS.

Lupus Erythematosus and Wegener's Granulomatosis.   Patients with lupus erythematosus or Wegener's granulomatosis sometimes may have diffuse pulmonary hemorrhage with an immunologic basis. The diagnosis of pulmonary hemorrhage should be considered in such patients with diffuse lung disease, but these patients also may have pulmonary edema or diffuse infection (Fig. 1.5).

Goodpasture's Syndrome.   In patients with Goodpasture's syndrome or rapidly progressive glomerulonephritis, pulmonary hemorrhage is not uncommon and can be suspected with the appearance of diffuse lung disease. In some patients, particularly those with Goodpasture's syndrome, pulmonary disease may precede recognition of the renal disease.

Diffuse Lung Disease

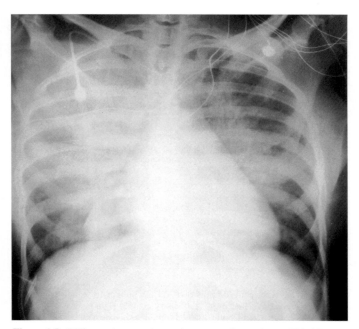

Figure 1.5. Diffuse pulmonary hemorrhage secondary to lupus. This 30-year-old woman with known lupus developed fairly extensive bilateral alveolar infiltrates that proved to be diffuse pulmonary hemorrhage. This is indistinguishable from pulmonary edema.

Idiopathic Pulmonary Hemosiderosis. Idiopathic pulmonary hemosiderosis is a rare disease. Though it occurs primarily in children, it can cause diffuse pulmonary hemorrhage. Many believe this is a form fruste of Goodpasture's disease.

Diffuse Infection

Most pulmonary infections are not diffuse in nature; rather, they are characterized by focal opacities. Certain types of infection can be quite diffuse, however. Causes of diffuse infection include:

> 1. *Pneumocystis carinii* pneumonia.
> 2. Certain viral pneumonias.
> 3. Aspiration pneumonia.
> 4. Bacterial pneumonia, especially that from *Legionella* sp.

Pneumocystic Carinii *Pneumonia.* *Pneumocystis carinii* pneumonia probably is the most common pneumonia to cause diffuse lung disease, at least among urban populations in which AIDS and other syndromes causing immunologic suppression are fairly common. *P. carinii* usually causes a pneumonia that appears to be interstitial on chest films but, occasionally, can appear to be a diffuse air-space infection (Fig 1.6). In this instance, it is difficult to distinguish from cardiac pulmonary edema, because many of these chronically ill patients, particularly patients with AIDS, also have associated cardiac disease.

Viral Pneumonia. Viral pneumonias usually cause a patchy nonsegmental or a lobar pneumonia that cannot be distinguished from bacterial pneumonias. Some viral pneumonias, however, may be very diffuse and quite acute. Influenza is one of these. Pneumonia is not common in patients with influenza, but it may occur in patients suffering from either epidemic or sporadic influenza and, in such people, is often life-threatening.

Varicella may cause diffuse pneumonia in patients with immunocompromise and even in normal hosts. Most community-acquired viral pneumonias do not cause diffuse disease.

Aspiration. Aspiration usually causes patchy focal opacities, which are recognized as patchy pneumonia (Fig. 1.3A). In some cases, however, aspiration causes a very diffuse pattern that cannot be distinguished from that of cardiac pulmonary edema. Many cases of aspiration cause focal pulmonary edema, because the aspirated fluid may contain only sterile gastric contents with a large amount of gastric acid. The low pH of the gastric acid produces the pulmonary edema, and though usually focal, this edema can be quite diffuse if the aspiration is extensive.

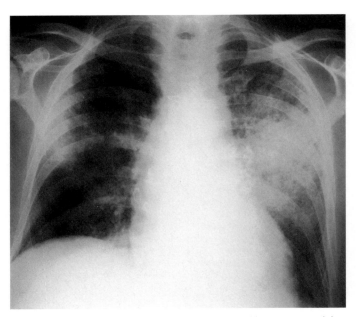

Figure 1.6. Pneumocystis pneumonia. This 36-year-old man was receiving immunosuppressive therapy for glioblastoma multiforme. Diffuse alveolar lung disease is present (greater on the left than the right) that proved to be pneumocystis pneumonia.

In patients with this type of aspiration, pulmonary edema may clear very rapidly (1–2 days). Many cases of aspiration, however, proceed to bacterial pneumonia or diffuse ARDS. It is difficult to tell when aspiration pneumonia ceases and ARDS begins. That the patchy nature of the pneumonia disappears and the consolidation in the lungs becomes quite homogeneous and diffuse may be one clue (Fig. 1.3).

Bacterial Pneumonia.   Bacterial pneumonias rarely are diffuse. Most bacteria involve only focal portions of the lungs, and even if they involve a large amount of one or both lungs, they still are focal diseases (i.e., "extensive localized" disease). Occasionally, however, a bacterial pneumonia may be diffuse. *Legionella* sp. frequently are responsible. Like diffuse viral pneumonia or aspiration, this type of pneumonia often proceeds rapidly to ARDS. All diffuse pneumonias initially cannot be distinguished from pulmonary edema.

Chronic Alveolar Lung Disease

Chronic alveolar lung disease is uncommon. Chronic diffuse alveolar disease is very uncommon.

Alveolar Proteinosis.   Alveolar proteinosis is a chronic alveolar disease of unknown origin that often has the appearance of pulmonary edema (Fig. 1.7). In this disease, alveoli are filled with hyaline material and treated with pulmonary

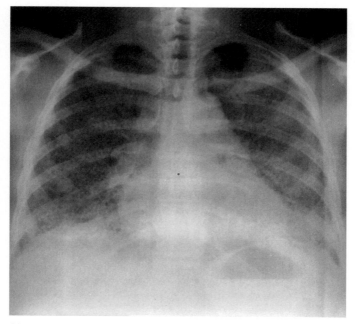

Figure 1.7. Alveolar proteinosis. This 36-year-old man had chronic alveolar infiltrates that proved to be pulmonary alveolar proteinosis.

lavage. After several years of repeated lavage, as the duration of disease process is more prolonged, it may appear less purely alveolar and somewhat more interstitial.

Alveolar proteinosis usually is primary, but it also may be secondary to other diseases. Lymphoproliferative malignancies may be complicated by alveolar proteinosis. This usually is confused with chronic infection when first encountered, but the chronic nature and lack of response to antibiotics often are suggestive of the diagnosis.

In patients with an acute, extensive exposure to silica (e.g., sand blasters), silicoproteinosis may be a manifestation of this exposure. Silicosis usually takes decades to appear, but silicoproteinosis may only take several years.

Alveolar proteinosis is sometimes complicated by infection with an unusual organism: *Nocardia* sp. Cavitary disease in patients with alveolar proteinosis is suggestive of the diagnosis. Other organisms that rarely may complicate alveolar proteinosis are the atypical mycobacteria.

Diffuse Bronchoalveolar Carcinoma. Bronchoalveolar carcinoma probably involves two different diseases. The solitary type is a peripheral nodule in the lung. It grows slowly and has a very favorable prognosis when resected.

The diffuse type is more unusual and presents as alveolar opacities throughout both lung fields. These usually are not coalescent but present as multiple acinar nodules or pulmonary rosettes (Fig. 1.8). This type of bronchoalveolar

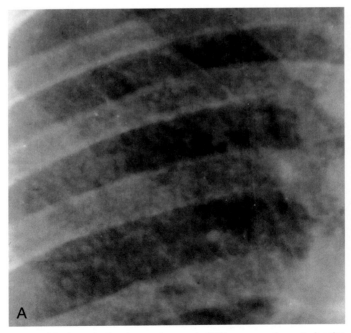

Figure 1.8. Bronchoalveolar carcinoma. **A.** Diffuse noncoalescent alveolar nodules in a 50-year-old man. **B.** A 60-year-old woman with diffuse noncoalescent nodules but one patchy area in the right upper lobe.

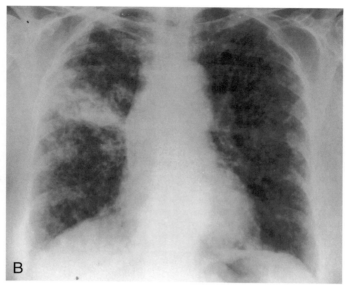

Figure 1.8. (*continued*)

carcinoma occasionally is preceded by a large, patchy consolidation in the lung (Fig. 1.8*B*) or a very coalescent lobar infiltrate. The diagnosis of diffuse bronchoalveolar carcinoma is a death knell; patients with this diagnosis seldom survive longer 2 years.

A metastatic tumor, usually from the breast, occasionally may mimic bronchoalveolar carcinoma radiographically and even histopathologically.

Hypersensitivity Lung and Desquamative Interstitial Pneumonitis. Two diseases that usually appear to be interstitial lung disease—hypersensitivity lung and desquamative interstitial pneumonitis (DIP)—also sometimes present as an alveolar disease. These diseases usually are quite diffuse, may exhibit a combination of interstitial and air-space disease, and are discussed in greater detail in the following section.

INTERSTITIAL LUNG DISEASE

The term *interstitial lung disease* implies involvement of the pulmonary interstitium by some infiltrative process. If alveolar disease is contrasted with interstitial disease, the characteristics of interstitial lung disease include:

1. Interstitial disease is noncoalescent and exhibits a pattern of discrete, small markings in both lungs.
2. Interstitial disease usually is diffuse; if not, it usually is symmetrical. Certain diseases involve the lower lung zones primarily and others the upper lung zones.

Diffuse Lung Disease

3. The patterns created by interstitial disease usually are nodular, linear, or reticular.
4. Interstitial diseases usually are chronic.

Radiographic Patterns in Interstitial Lung Disease

Considering the many causes of interstitial lung disease, it is useful to categorize them on the basis of their radiographic pattern. Most diseases involve the lungs in a fairly consistent (though not absolutely consistent) radiographic pattern. If you recognize the pattern, then you frequently can establish a rather accurate diagnosis.

Useful divisions of these patterns are nodular, reticular and linear groups. Nodular lung disease, of course, implies many nodules in the lungs. These nodules can be very tiny, like a grain of sand, or they can be larger, up to the size of a pea. Reticular disease exhibits a reticular (i.e., spider-web) or cystic pattern. In some cases, this pattern is very cystic and has been called a "honeycomb" pattern. Finally, linear disease exhibits Kerley lines. Kerley A lines are long lines radiating from the hila. Kerley B lines are small short lines occurring laterally at the lung bases, and Kerley C lines are a reticular pattern. Thus, on a film with a linear pattern, one also may recognize a reticular pattern, but if Kerley lines are recognized, they should take precedence and this pattern be recognized as linear and not reticular.

Linear Lung Diseases

Few diseases cause a linear interstitial pattern. Common ones include:

1. Interstitial pulmonary edema.
2. Interstitial infection, especially with *P. carinii.*
3. Lymphangitic carcinomatosis.

Interstitial Pulmonary Edema.   Alveolar pulmonary edema has already been described as a classic manifestation of heart failure. Alveolar edema always starts in the interstitium, but occasionally, one encounters a patient at the phase in which all pulmonary edema is interstitial and no alveolar edema is seen. This phase can occur in any patient with heart failure and is recognized by a linear interstitial pattern with loss of distinctness of the pulmonary vasculature (Fig 1.9). For some reason, it is commonly seen in patients with AIDS who also have heart failure and, of course, is difficult to distinguish from *P. carinii* pneumonia. If one suspects the cause of interstitial lung disease to be interstitial edema, it can be proven readily by diuresis with subsequent clearing of the interstitial pattern.

Interstitial Infection.   The major cause of interstitial pneumonia encountered in hospitals with a fairly large population of patients with immunosuppression is *P. carinii* pneumonia. This pneumonia may cause diffuse alveolar consolidation or sometimes focal alveolar consolidation, but the common pattern is diffuse interstitial pneumonia, often with a linear configuration (Fig. 1.10) but occasionally with a nodular or reticular pattern. As mentioned, interstitial pneumonia is difficult to distinguish from interstitial pulmonary edema. Clinical history may help in separating these two causes of the linear pattern. Diuresis and

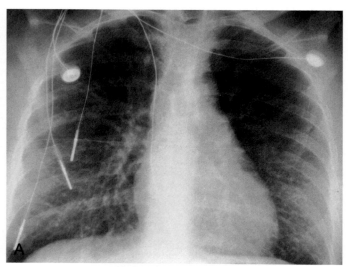

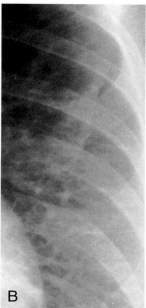

Figure 1.9. Interstitial pulmonary edema. **A.** A linear pattern is seen throughout both lungs and is associated with a prominent vascular pattern. **B.** Close-up view.

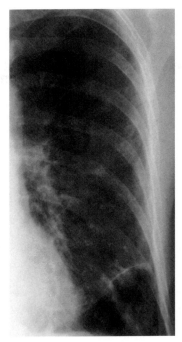

Figure 1.10. Pneumocystis pneumonia. A linear interstitial pattern is present in this 28-year-old man with AIDS and pneumocystis pneumonia.

follow-up chest films also are useful in distinguishing pulmonary edema from *P. carinii* pneumonia. This type of pneumonia will not disappear with diuresis.

Viral and mycoplasmal pneumonias often are typified as being interstitial. In our practice, that is not common, though it occasionally does occur (particularly with viral pneumonia). Viral and mycoplasmal pneumonias generally take other patterns. In most cases, they cannot be distinguished from bacterial pneumonia and cause lobar or patchy nonsegmental consolidation.

Other viral pneumonias such as cytomegalic virus (CMV) sometimes may cause an interstitial pattern, but these patterns usually are nodular. *Chlamydia* sp. sometimes may cause a linear interstitial pattern in infants.

Lymphagitic Carcinomatosis. Carcinoma can spread to the lung in several ways. Most metastatic carcinomas break out of the blood vessels in the lung and grow as a small, round nodule that pushes the alveoli aside and then becomes a well-circumscribed nodule in the interstitium. In some cases, metastatic tumor may invade the alveoli and cause an alveolar pattern in the lung. This is particularly true of breast carcinoma, but it may be seen with other types as well.

In other cases, the tumor spreads through the interlobular septa when it breaks out of the blood vessel. In this fashion, the tumor grows both in and around the

Diffuse Lung Disease

lymphatics, which also lie in the interlobular septa. This pattern of growth has led histopathologists to call this type of metastatic tumor "lymphagitic" (Fig. 1.11). Most tumors that metastasize to the lungs with a pattern of lymphangitic spread do so in a very diffuse fashion. It is unusual to see focal lymphangitic spread. Common tumors that produce lymphangitic spread are breast (the most common), lung, and two abdominal tumors—pancreatic and stomach—that commonly do not metastasize to the lung but, when they do, almost always spread in a lymphangitic fashion.

The diagnosis of lymphangitic tumor spread often can be established with a great deal of certainty. A chronic linear pattern generally is not suggestive of interstitial pulmonary edema or of interstitial infection, so one is left with only the diagnosis of lymphangitic carcinoma.

Reticular Interstitial Lung Disease

Reticular interstitial lung disease is recognized as a fine network of lines producing a series of tiny, polygonal spaces. Sometimes it also is recognized as a series of small cysts. Common causes of reticular interstitial disease include:

1. Collagen vascular disease.
2. Idiopathic pulmonary fibrosis (IPF).
3. Asbestosis.
4. End-stage lung.
5. Eosinophilic granuloma and lymphangiomyomatosis.

Collagen Vascular Disease.   All collagen vascular diseases involve the lung in a similar and characteristic fashion. The two most common collagen vascular diseases that cause lung disease are rheumatoid arthritis and scleroderma (i.e., progressive systemic sclerosis). Dermatomyositis, however, may give a very similar appearance. Lupus erythematosus ordinarily does not cause interstitial lung disease. Patients diagnosed with lupus who also have interstitial lung disease likely have a mixed connective tissue disorder or an overlap syndrome.

Early in the course of pulmonary involvement by collagen vascular disease, there may be an alveolar pattern in the involved area of lung (Fig. 1.12). This is quite unusual; a reticular interstitial pattern is much more common. Collagen vascular diseases characteristically involve the lung bases primarily—and often *only* the lung bases. In these cases, one may encounter a fine reticular pattern involving only lower 2 or 3 cm of lung (Fig. 1.13). In other cases, the entire lung may be involved, but these patients usually have a basilar predominance to the disease.

It is extremely rare for pulmonary involvement to be the initial finding in patients with collagen vascular disease. In most cases, patients will have been diagnosed with a collagen vascular disease in the past and only subsequently will interstitial lung disease develop. The interstitial disease frequently is quite indolent but occasionally may be rapidly progressive. At computed tomography (CT), the interstitial disease again has a basilar and often peripheral distribution.

Idiopathic Pulmonary Fibrosis.   Idiopathic pulmonary fibrosis probably is the most common diffuse interstitial disease encountered in daily practice. Histopathologists recognize a distinctive histopathologic pattern in IPF and most often term it *usual interstitial pneumonitis* (UIP). This is a disease of older patients and affects males more frequently than females. It usually progresses

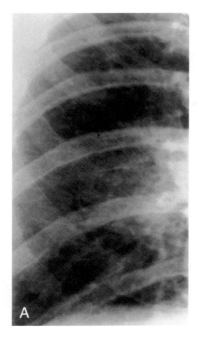

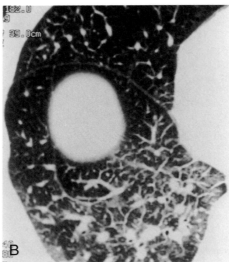

Figure 1.11. Lymphangitic spread of carcinoma. **A.** A diffuse linear pattern is seen throughout the visualized right lung. (The left lung was the same.) **B.** High-resolution CT scan in another patient shows characteristic filling of the interlobular septa with tumor.

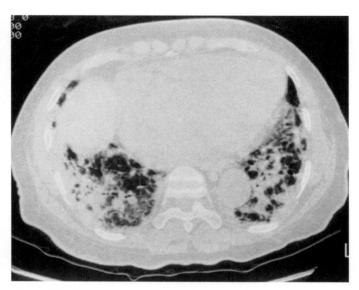

Figure 1.12. Dermatomyositis with alveolar disease at the bases. High-resolution CT scan shows a mixture of alveolar and reticular interstitial lung disease.

over time, either slowly or rapidly, but generally to a point at which it causes pulmonary failure and death. If this disease has a short, fulminant course, it often has a histopathologic pattern of acute interstitial pneumonitis rather than the more common UIP. Most patients with IPF do not have acute interstitial pneumonitis but the more prolonged variant of this disease. Acute interstitial pneumonitis was formerly known as the Hamman-Rich syndrome.

Another histopathologic pattern of IPF is DIP. This is reported as more commonly than UIP having an alveolar component or as being completely alveolar. Many believe that DIP and UIP are variants of the same disease process and that the degree of alveolar involvement merely reflects the stage at which the disease is encountered. Recent reports suggest that DIP is a manifestation of cigarette smoking. DIP reportedly responds better to steroid therapy, but steroid therapy usually is tried in both diseases (with unpredictable results).

Another disease process that cannot be distinguished on chest films from UIP and that sometimes is confused histopathologically with UIP is bronchiolitis obliterans organizing pneumonia. This is extremely steroid responsive, and it may account for some of the very good responses of DIP and UIP to steroids in earlier reports, before the recent description of bronchiolitis obliterans organizing pneumonia.

The radiographic pattern of IPF, regardless of its histopathologic pattern, is one of basilar interstitial lung disease or peripheral interstitial lung disease or of diffuse interstitial lung disease (Fig. 1.14), any of which cannot be distinguished from collagen vascular disease either on plain films or on high-resolution CT scans. There probably is some form of relationship between the collagen vascular diseases and IPF, because both have immunologic origins and many pa-

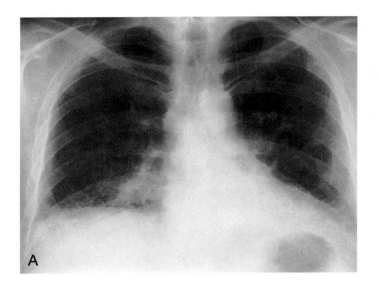

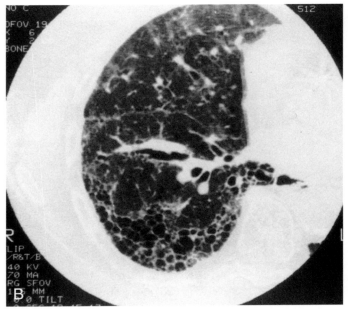

Figure 1.13. Scleroderma with reticular lung disease. **A.** This 40-year-old woman had mild reticular lung disease most clearly marked in the lung bases. **B.** High-resolution CT scan of a 44-year-old woman shows the reticular characteristics of this disease.

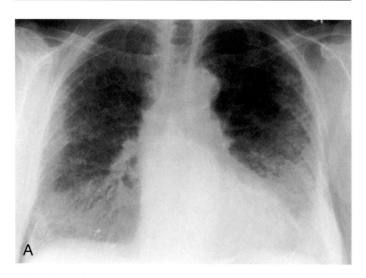

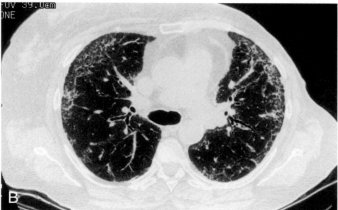

Figure 1.14. Idiopathic pulmonary fibrosis. **A.** This 65-year-old man had diffuse reticular lung disease. **B.** High-resolution CT scan of the same patient shows the peripheral nature of the reticular changes.

tients with IPF also have nonspecific circulating antibodies (e.g., rheumatoid factor, lupus antigens).

Asbestosis.   Asbestosis is the third reticular interstitial lung disease that causes basilar opacities (Fig. 1.15). This diagnosis usually can be established easily on the basis of patient history, because heavy exposure to asbestos particles is necessary for development of asbestosis. In addition, patients with asbestosis usu-

Diffuse Lung Disease

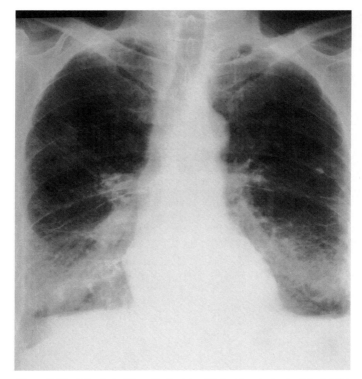

Figure 1.15. Asbestosis. The reticular interstitial pattern is most marked at the bases. Note also the asbestos-related pleural changes.

ally have asbestos-related pleural plaques; such plaques can occur in patients with only minimal asbestos exposure. Once a fairly common interstitial lung disease, asbestosis is very uncommon today. The manufacturing community is aware of the deleterious effects of asbestos on the lungs and has reduced the exposure of workers to these particles.

Asbestosis also may not be distinguishable from collagen vascular disease or IPF. The reticular interstitial pattern often is somewhat coarser than that encountered in patients IPF or collagen vascular disease, however. The diagnosis usually is established on the basis of the exposure history.

Patients exposed to asbestos have a statistically significant increased incidence of malignancy, particularly lung carcinoma and pleural mesothelioma.

End-Stage Lung. The term *end-stage lung* is given to patients with long-standing lung disease who, at biopsy or autopsy, show only severe pulmonary fibrosis and diffuse honeycombing of the lungs. Many diseases that might be diagnosed readily early in the course of disease only show fibrosis later in the disease. These diseases include sarcoidosis, eosinophilic granuloma, IPF, hypersensitivity lung, and occasionally other lung diseases. End-stage lung usually manifests as a coarse, very diffuse reticular pattern throughout both lungs with fairly large reticular or cystic spaces.

Eosinophilic Granuloma and Lymphangiomyomatosis. The four diseases discussed so far are the usual causes of reticular interstitial lung disease. Eosinophilic granuloma (i.e., histiocytosis X) and lymphangiomyomatosis are interstitial diseases that are marked by preservation of lung volume, whereas most restrictive lung diseases are marked by loss of lung volume. Both diseases produce cystic changes in the lung later in the course of disease that create a characteristic cystic or reticular pattern (Fig. 1.16).

Eosinophilic granuloma usually involves the upper lobes much more than the lower lobes. It is a disease of young patients (in their twenties and thirties), usually of males, and generally is slowly progressive. It is remotely related to eosinophilic granuloma of bone, because approximately 5% of patients with eosinophilic granuloma of the lung also have eosinophilic granuloma of bone. The diagnosis is unlikely without a patient history of smoking. Considering that there is no known cure, lung transplantation often is required as treatment. Steroids have been used in therapy, but patient response is poor.

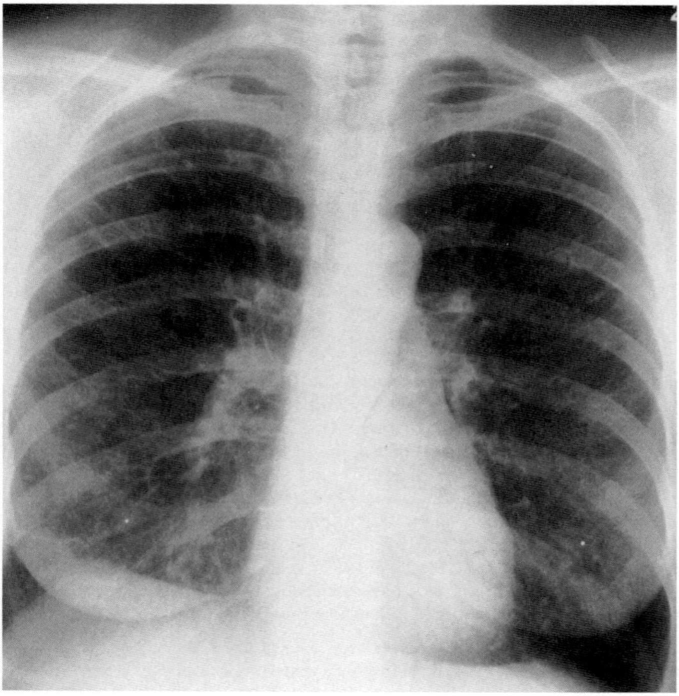

Figure 1.16. Lymphangiomyomatosis. Diffuse reticular interstitial disease and mild hyperinflation in a 36-year-old woman with lymphangiomyomatosis.

Lymphangiomyomatosis is another rare disease that is seen in females and, when it involves the lungs, cannot be distinguished histopathologically from tuberous sclerosis. Like eosinophilic granuloma, lymphangiomyomatosis causes mild hyperinflation of the lungs, cystic changes of the lungs, and a reticular or sometimes nodular interstitial lung disease. This disease process frequently requires lung transplantation as well. High-resolution CT scans are extremely useful in establishing the diagnosis in either disease.

Sarcoidosis.   Sarcoidosis, which is nodular during the early stages, may cause cystic changes in the lung and a reticular appearance. Unlike the eosinophilic granuloma and lymphangiomyomatosis, however, patients with sarcoidosis usually have low lung volumes (unless they have associated emphysema).

Nodular Interstitial Lung Disease

Nodular interstitial lung disease produces a pattern of multiple, tiny, well-defined nodular densities. The nodules may vary in size but usually range from 1 to 2 mm. These nodules should be quite regular as well. Irregular nodules are suggestive of the acinar pattern associated with alveolar disease and particularly bronchoalveolar carcinoma.

There are many causes of nodular interstitial lung disease, but the patient history often allows the proper disease process to be identified. Some common causes include:

1. Metastatic tumor.
2. Silicosis and benign pneumoconioses.
3. Sarcoidosis.
4. Hypersensitivity lung.
5. Toxic lung disease.
6. Infection, especially miliary tuberculosis.
7. Eosinophilic granuloma and lymphangiomyomatosis.

Metastatic Tumor.   Metastatic tumor has several patterns in the lung, and it may metastasize with an alveolar or a lymphangitic pattern. Most metastatic tumors are nodular, however, because they most often grow in a concentric, radial fashion. The resulting nodular metastases seen in most tumors are not very numerous, numbering only in the tens to hundreds, and are fairly large. Therefore, they can be recognized readily as metastatic tumors, and the differential diagnosis is one of multiple pulmonary nodules rather than interstitial lung disease.

Occasionally, metastatic tumors can create multiple tiny nodules throughout the lung fields and have the appearance of interstitial disease (Fig. 1.17). The primary tumors most likely to do this are thyroid tumors, melanoma, and breast tumors. These tumors often cause nodules that are larger than the usual nodular interstitial pattern (diameter, 3–4 mm). These might be designated "medium-size" interstitial nodules. Metastatic tumors are one of the few entities that cause medium-size nodules (Fig. 1.17); silicosis is another (Fig. 1.18).

Silicosis and Benign Pneumoconioses.   Whereas asbestosis causes a basilar reticular pattern, silicosis causes a nodular pattern involving the upper lung fields. The nodules can vary in size but usually are quite small and often referred as to "sand-like" (Fig. 1.18*B*). Upper lung field involvement is characteristic and consistent in this disease and often is suggestive of the diagnosis. Con-

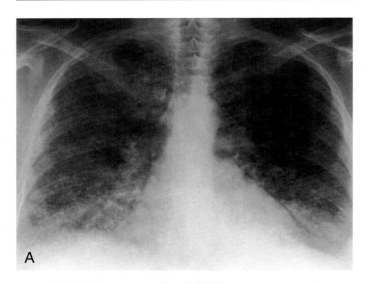

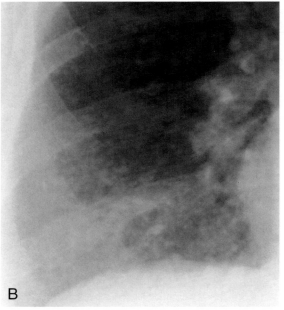

Figure 1.17. Metastatic tumor. **A.** Metastatic melanoma. **B.** Metastatic thyroid carcinoma. Note the fine nodular interstitial pattern in parts A and B.

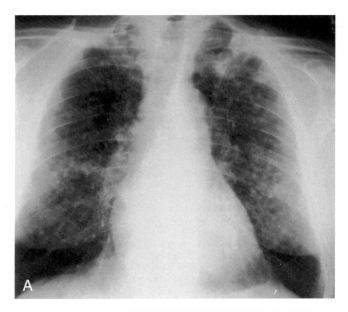

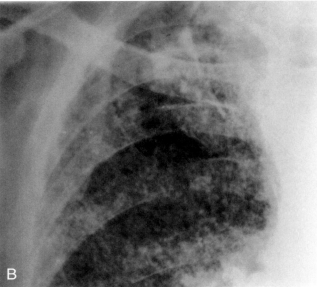

Figure 1.18. Silicosis. **A.** This 56-year-old man had multiple medium-size nodules with an upper lobe predominance. Note the small conglomerate nodule in the left upper lobe. Nodules are characteristic of silicosis. **B.** This 63-year-old-man has silicosis, a conglomerate nodule, and extensive small interstitial nodules with an upper lobe predominance.

25

glomerate masses are nodular areas of coalescent opacity that usually occur in the upper or middle lobes. They are another characteristic of silicosis and are strongly suggestive of this disease (Fig. 1.18). These conglomerate masses, however, may be confused with other lung masses such as bronchogenic carcinoma or tuberculosis.

Silicosis is caused by exposure to sand, and such exposure occurs in several occupations. Coal mining and sand blasting are the best known. Potters, steel workers, quarry workers, and other industrial workers may be exposed to silica as well. Among coal miners, this is sometimes termed *coal worker's pneumoconiosis*. It probably is possible for those exposed only to carbon (i.e., coal) to develop nodular interstitial lung disease, but most cases of coal worker's disease probably result from exposure to silica (i.e., sandstone) mixed in with the coal.

The benign pneumoconioses are those that develop pulmonary nodules secondary to exposure to nonfibrogenic dusts. They are called "benign," because these dusts, unlike silica and asbestos, do not cause true fibrosis in the lungs. The benign pneumoconioses include exposure to iron, aluminum, and various other metals. Silicosis and asbestosis create fibrosis in the lung by producing a local immunologic reaction that results in interstitial fibrosis and therefore are more harmful to the patient. The benign pneumoconioses are generalized, however, and do not have the upper lobe predominance of silicosis or the lower lobe predominance of asbestosis.

Sarcoidosis.   A disease of unknown cause, sarcoidosis can create several patterns in the lung. Early in the development of many cases, a fine, nodular interstitial pattern is present that usually involves the upper lung fields more than the lower lung fields. A major clue to the diagnosis of sarcoidosis is lymphadenopathy, which can occur at all stages of the disease but particularly early in the course. It also is fairly common to have patchy nodules and infiltrates, which appear to be alveolar, early in the disease. Histopathologically, these are not truly alveolar, but it probably is appropriate for radiologists to call them alveolar because they cannot be distinguished from other alveolar diseases. Late in the course of disease, a cystic or reticular pattern is fairly common.

Another characteristic of sarcoidosis is a mid-lung-zone distribution, which is virtually pathognomonic of sarcoidosis. This distribution occasionally may occur with the nodular interstitial pattern, but it is more common late in the course of disease (with midzone scarring).

Hypersensitivity Lung.   Hypersensitivity pneumonitis or extrinsic allergic alveolitis sometimes may cause an alveolar pattern but usually causes a fine nodular pattern that is diffuse and has no upper or lower lobe predilection (Fig. 1.19). Hypersensitivity pneumonitis can occur secondary to inhalation of various allergens. These inhalational diseases usually are known by occupation or the source of the organic material being inhaled. Included in this group are farmer's lung, pigeon breeder's disease, humidifier lung, byssinosis (i.e., cotton fibers), bagassosis (i.e., sugar cane), maple bark disease, mushroom worker's disease, and others. The common denominator among these various inhalational diseases are microorganisms, which usually are thermophylic actinomycetes, *Microspora faenii,* or *Aspergillus* sp.. Beryllium is a metal that also causes inhalational hypersensitivity (Fig. 1.19).

Hypersensitivity pneumonitis also can be caused by bloodborne allergens (usually drugs). Various drugs, including such simple ones as antibiotics or di-

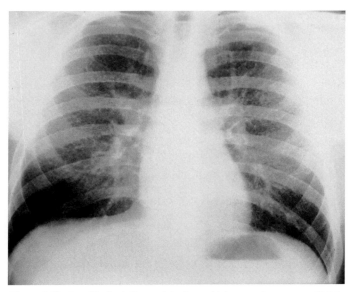

Figure 1.19. Berylliosis. A fine nodular interstitial pattern is present, which is characteristic of hypersensitivity lung disease. The causative allergen in this instance was beryllium.

uretics, may cause hypersensitivity lung; the most common drugs are chemotherapeutic agents such as methotrexate, 5-fluorouracil, and so on. In patients receiving this type of chemotherapy, it often is difficult to distinguish between diffuse infection and a drug reaction in the lung.

Amniodorone is a cardiac drug that also may cause hypersensitivity lung. Hypersensitivity lung usually produces multiple tiny nodules, which are scattered diffusely throughout the lungs and have no predilection for the upper or lower lobes. Histopathologically, these nodules are granulomas.

Toxic Lung Disease. Hypersensitivity lung implies an idiosyncratic, allergic reaction to a drug or an inhalational agent. In some cases, however, a predictive pulmonary reaction from certain amounts of a drug or exposure to certain agents occurs. These patients have a toxic rather than an allergic reaction. The radiographic pattern is quite similar to that of hypersensitivity lung disease.

Among the drugs that cause a toxic reaction are some chemotherapeutic agents, particularly busulfan. Paraquat, which is an insecticide, also may cause nodular interstitial lung disease that, with significant exposure, may progress to ARDS.

Inhalational gases that cause interstitial lung disease likely are those from acids, such as sulfuric acid, hydrochloric acid, and nitric acid (as produced in silo filler's disease). These agents most commonly cause an acute alveolar reaction, but long-term exposure can lead to nodular interstitial lung disease.

27

Diffuse Lung Disease

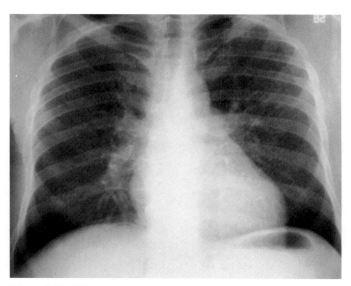

Figure 1.20. Miliary tuberculosis in a normal host. Fine nodular interstitial disease is seen in this nonimmunosuppressed patient that proved to be miliary tuberculosis.

Nodular Interstitial Infection. Few infections create a nodular interstitial pattern, but most important of these is miliary tuberculosis (Fig. 1.20). This condition usually occurs during primary exposure in a patient with no immune defense, and the tuberculous organisms spread in a metastatic fashion throughout all organs of the body. In the lungs, this manifests as multiple nodules. Rarely, one may see overflow into the alveoli with a mixed interstitial and alveolar pattern, similar to pulmonary edema, as the disease becomes more advanced.

Just as tuberculosis can create a miliary pattern, so can various fungal diseases. The most common are epidemic histoplasmosis and coccidioidomycosis.

Cytomegalovirus causes a diffuse infection that may be occult and not seen on the chest film of patients with immunosuppression. Sometimes, however, it may be seen on chest films as a fine nodular pattern in the lungs.

Eosinophilic Granuloma and Lymphangiomyomatosis. Eosinophilic granuloma can present as either nodular or reticular lung disease. It characteristically involves the upper lung fields much more than the lower lung fields. Lymphangiomyomatosis, which is another disease of unknown cause that occurs in women, also can present as a nodular interstitial pattern, though the pattern more typically is reticular.

After learning to recognize the three patterns—nodular, reticular, and linear—you you can be reasonably accurate when identifying the nature of various interstitial lung diseases. You should be able to "get in right the ball park" 75% to 85% of the time.

Diffuse Lung Disease

SUGGESTED READINGS

Aberle DR, Wiener-Kronish P, Webb WR, Matthay MA. Hydrostatic versus increased permeability pulmonary edema: diagnosis based on radiographic criteria in critically ill patients. Radiology 1988;168:73–79.

Albelda SM, Gefter WB, Epstein DM, Miller WT. Diffuse pulmonary hemorrhage: a review and classification. Radiology 1985;154:289–297.

Bergin CJ, Muller NL. CT of interstitial lung disease: a diagnostic approach. AJR 1987;148:8–15.

Crow J, Slavin G, Kreel L. Pulmonary metastases: a pathologic and radiologic study. Cancer 1981;47:2395–2602.

Feigen DS. Interstitial lung diseases: new perspectives. Radiol Clin North Am 1983;2l:683–697.

Felson B. The interstitium in chest roentgenology. Philadelphia: WB Saunders, 1973:329–429.

Felson B. The roentgen diagnosis of disseminated pulmonary alveolar diseases. Semin Roentgenol 1967;2:3–21.

Freundlich IM. Alveolar consolidation. In: Freundlich IM, Bragg DG, eds. A radiologic approach to diseases of the chest. Baltimore: Williams & Wilkins, 1992:72–82.

McLoud TC, Carrington CB, Gaenseler EA. Diffuse infiltrative lung disease: a new scheme for description. Radiology 1983;149:353–363.

Meziane MA, Hruban RH, Zerhouni EA, et al. High resolution CT of the lung parenchyma with pathologic correlation. Radiographics 1988;8:27–54.

Miller WT, Husted J, Freiman D, Atkinson B, Pietra G. Bronchioloalveolar carcinoma: two clinical entities with one pathologic diagnosis. AJR 1978;130:867–875.

Milne ENC, Pistolesi M, Miniati M, Giuntini CC. The radiologic distinction of cardiogenic and noncardiogenic edema. AJR 1985;144:879–894.

Mueller N. Interstitial lung disease. In: Freundlich IM, Bragg, DG, eds. A radiologic approach to diseases of the chest. Baltimore: Williams & Wilkins, 1992:127–138.

Prophet D. Primary pulmonary histiocytosis-X. Clin Chest Med 1982;3:643–653.

Scadding JG, Mitchel DN, eds. Sarcoidosis. London: Chapman and Hall Medical, 1985:101–180.

Trapnell DH. The radiological appearance of lymphangitic carcinomatosis of the lung. Thorax 1964;19:2551–2560.

Focal Interstitial Lung Disease

2

Focal interstitial lung disease is not common—if we classify interstitial disease involving the bases or the apices symmetrically as a diffuse lung disease. Even with this definition, however, focal interstitial lung disease still occasionally occurs.

CAUSES

Certain processes can involve the interstitium of the lung in a focal fashion. Though uncommon, they include:

1. Lymphangitic carcinomatosis.
2. Interstitial infection, especially pneumocystis pneumonia.
3. Bronchiectasis.

Lymphangitic Carcinomatosis

In most instances, lymphangitic carcinomatosis is a diffuse process (see Chapter 1). Occasionally, however, lymphangitic carcinomatosis may involve primarily one lung or a focal portion of one lung (Fig. 2.1). The malignancies that often cause lymphangitic carcinomatosis occur in the breast, pancreas, stomach, and the lung itself. Any of these diseases may sometimes be focal—especially lung carcinoma, which may spread directly from the primary tumor to the surrounding lung via the lymphatic vessels. Rarely, other malignancies may involve the lungs in a lymphangitic fashion.

Interstitial Infection

Pulmonary infection generally appears as alveolar disease, but if the infection is interstitial, it usually presents in a diffuse fashion. Rarely, however, infection can appear as focal interstitial opacities. Pneumocystis and occasionally viral pneumonia also may present in this fashion (Fig. 2.2), as may neonatal chlamydial pneumonia.

Bronchiectasis

Though not an interstitial lung disease, bronchiectasis is often confused with interstitial lung disease. Bronchiectasis refers to an irreversible dilatation of the bronchi, usually secondary to infection. This infection may be an acute pneumonia that is treated incompletely or repeated bouts of pneumonia in the same location (as in right middle lobe syndrome). Some patients have immune defects or even impaired or mucociliary clearance; these patients are predisposed to recurrent pneumonias and subsequent bronchiectasis.

Bronchiectasis is caused by the following diseases:

1. Cystic fibrosis.
2. Allergic bronchopulmonary aspergillosis.
3. Immotile cilia (Kartagener's) syndrome.
4. Hypogamma globulinemia and other immune problems.
5. Swyer-James syndrome.

Focal Interstitial Lung Disease

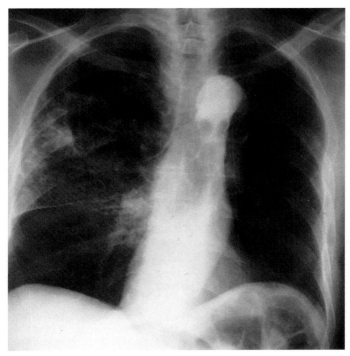

Figure 2.1. Lymphangitic spread of tumor. Lymphangitic spread of tumor is usually diffuse. In this 61-year-old man, however, the focal right upper lobe infiltrate was lymphangitic spread from pancreatic carcinoma.

Depending on the degree of bronchial dilatation, bronchiectasis produces various radiographic appearances. The earliest phase of bronchiectasis is cylindrical bronchiectasis. Ordinarily, bronchi become smaller as they branch. In cylindrical bronchiectasis, however, bronchi become slightly larger as they branch. There also tends to be loss of volume in the involved lung, with crowding of the bronchi. Cylindrical bronchiectasis usually is not visible on plain chest films, but it may be identified on high-resolution computed tomographic scans. In years past, cylindrical bronchiectasis was identified at bronchography.

As the bronchiectasis worsens, the bronchi becomes somewhat more dilated and tortuous. Like all tubular structures that elongate and dilate (e.g., vessels, esophagus, ureters), the bronchi become tortuous as the dilatation occurs. At this stage, the dilatation is *termed varicose bronchiectasis.*

The most advanced stage of bronchiectasis is cystic bronchiectasis, in which focal dilatation of the bronchial walls occurs between the cartilaginous rings. This results in multiple dilatations of the larger and midsize bronchi, which in

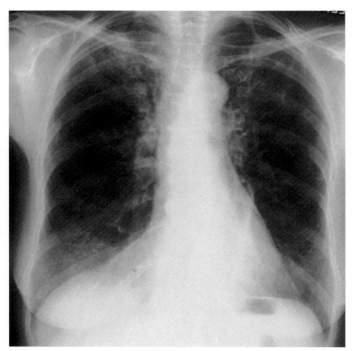

Figure 2.2. Pneumocystis pneumonia. This 43-year-old woman with AIDS had focal pneumocystis pneumonia involving the upper lobes. This may occur in patients receiving prophylactic pentamidine aerosal, as was the case in this patient.

turn results in a cystic appearance, with air (or sometimes air-fluid levels) in the dilated bronchi. Occasionally, these dilated bronchi can fill with fluid and appear as multiple, large nodules in the lung. The radiographic appearance of cystic bronchiectasis is often indistinguishable from that of reticular interstitial lung disease (Fig. 2.3).

Because bronchiectasis usually occurs secondary to infection, which also often has an obstruction associated with it, the bronchiectasis occurs in the localized area involved by the infection. Certain areas are more susceptible to the formation of bronchiectasis than others, however. The right middle lobe is the most susceptible; therefore, a specific name indicates chronic or repeated infections in this lobe: right middle lobe syndrome (Fig. 2.4). Usually, loss of volume is associated with severe cylindrical or cystic bronchiectasis. Chronic infections occur most commonly in the right middle lobe but can occur in any lobe. Thus, it is probably appropriate to designate another lobe having this ap-

Focal Interstitial Lung Disease

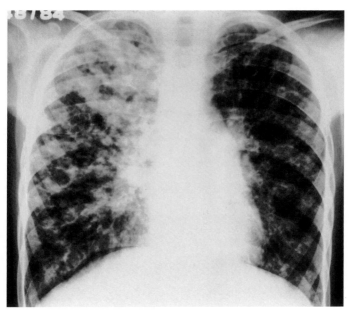

Figure 2.3. Extensive bronchiectasis and cystic fibrosis. Cystic (ring) shadows are present diffusely throughout both lungs but are marked in the upper lobes—particularly on the right side—in this 23-year-old man with cystic fibrosis. These cystic areas represent bronchiectasis; many of the bronchiectatic areas are filled with fluid.

pearance as the "right middle lobe syndrome in the [appropriate] lobe." After the right middle lobe, bronchiectasis occurs most commonly in the lingula and then in the lower lobes. Bronchiectasis occurring in an upper lobe of a normal patient is usually secondary to previous tuberculosis.

An increasingly recognized cause of bronchiectasis is infection with various atypical mycobacterial organisms (also called anonymous mycobacteria or non-tuberculous mycobacteria) (Fig. 2.5). *Mycobacterium avium-intracellulare* or *M. kansasii* are the most common atypical mycobacteria to cause bronchiectasis, but other mycobacterial organisms can cause the same picture. In these diseases, bronchiectasis is more common in the upper lobes. Bronchiectasis can occur in any lobe, however, and is frequently multilobar.

Cystic fibrosis, allergic bronchopulmonary aspergillosis, immotile cilia (Kartagener's) syndrome, and hypogammaglobulinemia are diseases associated with impaired immunity, and they usually lead to very extensive bilateral bronchiectasis. This bronchiectasis may be worse in one or several localized areas but is usually quite extensive (Fig. 2.5). Diffuse bronchiectasis is suggestive

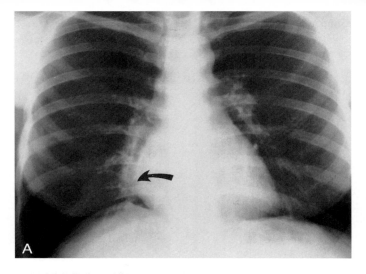

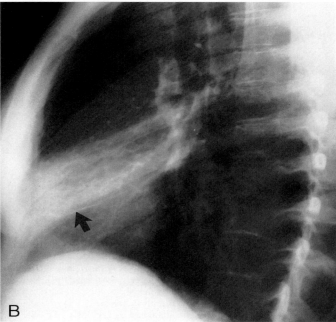

Figure 2.4. Right middle lobe bronchiectasis (right middle lobe syndrome). In this 29-year-old woman with hypogammaglobulinemia, chronic bronchiectasis of the right middle lobe (*arrow*) was present on the posteroanterior (**A**) and lateral (**B**) films. Right middle lobe syndrome is usually associated with bronchiectasis, atelectasis, or both.

34

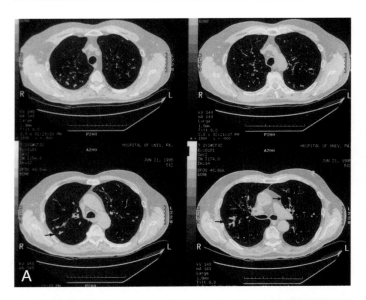

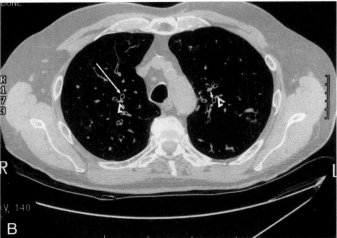

Figure 2.5. Infection with Mycobacterium avium-intracellulare causing diffuse bronchiectasis. **A.** This 60-year-old man had bronchiectasis (*arrows*) scattered throughout multiple areas. **B.** On this enlarged view, the bronchi (*closed arrows*) are larger than the vessels (*open arrows*).

Focal Interstitial Lung Disease

of one of these syndromes, and the diagnosis is frequently established on the basis of a careful patient history.

Cystic Fibrosis

Cystic fibrosis characteristically causes bilateral, extensive, upper lobe bronchiectasis. Thus, the diagnosis of cystic fibrosis can be considered when this pattern is encountered.

Allergic Bronchopulmonary Aspergillosis

Allergic bronchopulmonary aspergillosis occurs almost invariably in patients with asthma. It is associated with blood eosinophilia and is marked by filling of the dilated bronchi with inspissated mucus rather than air. Bronchiectasis in patients with allergic bronchopulmonary aspergillosis tends to be centrally located.

Immotile Cilia (Kartagener's) Syndrome

Approximately half of all patients with immotile cilia syndrome have situs inversus; thus, situs inversus with bronchiectasis is strongly suggestive of this diagnosis. These patients also have chronic sinusitis, as do many of the other patients who are immunologically impaired.

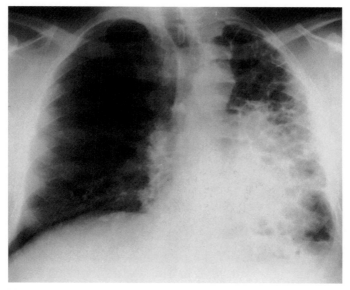

Figure 2.6. Diffuse bronchiectasis in the left lung secondary to Swyer-James syndrome. This 54-year-old woman had chronic bronchiectasis in the left lung as a result of neonatal infection (Swyer-James syndrome).

Focal Interstitial Lung Disease

Swyer-James Syndrome

Bronchiectasis that extensively involves one lung is suggestive of the diagnosis of Swyer-James syndrome (Fig. 2.6). Swyer-James syndrome occurs after neonatal infection (probably bronchiolitis), and it results in a small lung with hypoplasia of the pulmonary artery, air trapping, and usually bronchiectasis.

SUGGESTED READINGS

Barliner AF, Bardana EL. Bronchiectasis: update on an orphan disease. Am Rev Respir Dis 1988;137:969–978.

Bertolsen S, Struve-Christensen E, Aasted A, Sparup C. Isolated middle lobe atelectasis: etiology, pathogenesis, and treatment of the so-called middle lobe syndrome. Thorax 1980;35:449–452.

Fernald GW, Boat TF. Cystic fibrosis: overview. Semin Roentgenol 1987;22:87–96.

Libshitz HI, North LB. Pulmonary metastases. Radiol Clin North Am 1982;20:437–451.

Naidich DP, McCauley D, Khouri NF, Stitik EP, Siegelman SS. Computed tomography of bronchiectasis. J Comput Assist Tomogr 1983;6:437–444.

Focal Alveolar Infiltrates: Solitary or Multiple

3

Air-space (i.e., alveolar) disease was defined in Chapter 1. The radiographic appearance changes slightly, however, when focal alveolar disease is considered:

1. Focal density in the lung usually has irregular or "fluffy" margins. A focal alveolar density usually is confluent and appears to be solid and dense.
2. The silhouette sign and air bronchogram frequently are present, thereby indicating fluid-filled alveolar spaces and patent bronchi.
3. The distribution of the disease may be lobar or segmental, or it may be patchy and follow no anatomic boundaries.
4. Most alveolar diseases are acute (e.g., pneumonia), but there are several interesting chronic alveolar infiltrates. Sometimes, these infiltrates are cavitary, and cavitation may help to establish a specific diagnosis.

CAUSES

Causes of focal alveolar infiltrates include:

1. Infection.
   A. Bacterial pneumonia.
   B. Viral and mycoplasmal pneumonia.
   C. Aspiration.
   D. Tuberculosis.
   E. Atypical mycobacterial infection.
   F. Fungal infections.
2. Tumor.
   A. Primary carcinoma, especially bronchoalveolar carcinoma.
   B. Lymphoma.
   C. Metastatic carcinoma.
3. Pulmonary infarction.
4. Radiation.
5. Vasculitis, especially Wegener's granulomatosis.
6. Chronic eosinophilic pneumonia and other eosinophilic lung diseases.
7. Bronchiolitis obliterans organizing pneumonia.

Infection

Bacterial Pneumonia

Bacterial pneumonia frequently causes lobar consolidation, but it also may cause patchy segmental or nonsegmental consolidation or involve multiple areas of the lung (Fig. 3.1). Certain organisms are likely to cause lobar consolidation and others a nonsegmental "bronchopneumonia" pattern, but the radiographic appearance provides only a small clue regarding the organism. Identification of the causative organism depends on the results of a smear or culture of the organism from the sputum.

Viral and Mycoplasmal Pneumonia

Just as bacterial pneumonia can cause a lobar, segmental, or nonsegmental pattern, so can viral and mycoplasmal pneumonia. Infection with these viral and my-

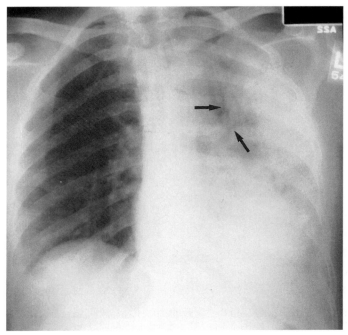

Figure 3.1. Pneumococcal pneumonia. Note the alveolar consolidation in the left upper and left lower lobes from pneumonia, which in this patient was caused by infection with pneumococcus. Note also the air bronchogram (*arrows*) in the left upper lobe.

coplasmal organisms, which frequently has been touted as interstitial pneumonia, usually causes a radiographic appearance that cannot be distinguished from that of bacterial pneumonia. In our experience, interstitial pneumonia caused by community-acquired viral or mycoplasmal organisms is a rather rare process.

Organisms Associated with Cavitation

Cavitation (i.e., lung abscess) may occur with pneumonia, and organisms such as *Staphylococcus*, *Pseudomonas*, and *Klebsiella* sp. are more likely to cause cavitation. When cavitation occurs, one of these organisms should be suspected, but cavitation can result from many organisms, including *Pneumococcus* sp. Lung abscess occasionally may cause thrombosis of the vessels supplying the lobe to the lung abscess and infarction of that lobe (Fig. 3.2). This development (i.e., pulmonary gangrene) usually is a serious, requiring surgical intervention to drain the lung abscess. *Klebsiella* sp. usually is the causative organism.

Rarely, pneumonias cause expansion of a lobe, which is indicated by bowing of the interlobar fissures. This is called a "drowned lobe" and most frequently results from *Klebsiella* sp.

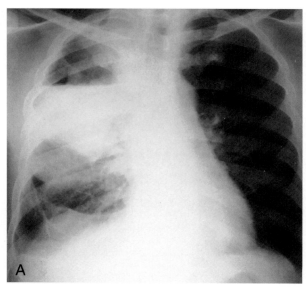

Figure 3.2. Lung abscess secondary to infection with *Klebsiella* sp. Posteroanterior (**A**) and lateral (**B**) films show consolidation of the right upper lobe with a large air-fluid level and a small right pleural effusion. This represents an extensive lung abscess, which in this 57-year-old man resulted from infection with *Klebsiella* sp. This patient probably had thrombosis of the right upper lobe vessels (gangrene).

Aspiration

Aspiration also frequently cannot be distinguished from the other causes of pneumonia. Aspiration may lead to a bacterial pneumonia if organisms are aspirated. If the aspirate is sterile, however, aspiration causes only focal pulmonary edema, which can clear rapidly because no true infection has occurred. Aspiration also may cause atelectasis, and it sometimes may cause a classic lobar pattern. The appearance of the consolidation usually is not helpful in predicting the course of the aspiration: it may go on to produce pneumonia; it may clear rapidly, because it produced only pulmonary edema; or particularly if extensive, it may proceed to adult respiratory distress syndrome.

The clue to aspiration as a cause for an alveolar infiltrate is that it frequently is bilateral or multilobar and usually involves the dependent areas of the lung (see Fig. 1.2*A*). In an upright patient, this is the lower lobe; in a supine patient in a hospital bed, this often involves the posterior segments of the lower lobes and the upper lobes.

Tuberculosis

Tuberculosis is unlike most other infectious diseases. It has both a primary and a reactivation phase.

Focal Alveolar Infiltrates

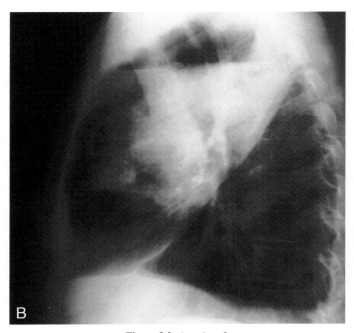

Figure 3.2. (*continued*)

In primary tuberculosis, the organism causes a local reaction in any area of the lung (usually a lower lobe). This area may be lobar or a patchy area of consolidation and not involve the entire lobe. If a good immune response is present, the local area of pneumonia gradually resolves in several weeks to months. The local process gradually shrinks to become a nodule, and the nodule then may disappear completely or become calcified (i.e., Ghon lesion).

As the disease progresses, organisms spread from the primary focus to the hilar and the mediastinal lymph nodes. If the immune response is good, the organism may go no further. In most cases, however, the organism disseminates to other areas of the body before the full immune response occurs. As a result, viable organisms spread to areas of high oxygen tension, such as the apices of the lungs, cortex of the long bones and kidneys, and the brain. The immune response then walls off these organisms, which then lie dormant for months to years and become activated again if the patient's immune system is compromised by old age, debility, or illness.

In addition to the primary focus in the lung, primary tuberculosis also may manifest, both clinically and radiographically, as mediastinal adenopathy, pleural effusion, or both. In countries where tuberculosis is common, primary tuberculosis mainly occurs in children. In the United States, primary tuberculosis mainly occurs in adults; few U.S. children are exposed to tuberculosis today.

Reactivation tuberculosis occurs when the immune system is compromised and, because they no longer are held in check by T-cell immunity, previously

Focal Alveolar Infiltrates

disseminated organisms begin to grow again. In the lungs, this produces an alveolar infiltration, usually in one or both of the upper lobes. This infiltration may be minimal or very extensive, and it may spread (i.e., bronchogenic spread) to involve much of both lungs. It often involves much of one lung and a small amount of the opposite lung, frequently the superior segment of the contralateral lower lobe, which is a pattern typical of bronchogenic spread. Cavitation in reactivation tuberculosis is extremely common (Fig. 3.3) but it does not occur in primary tuberculosis (Fig. 10.8).

If a poor immune response occurs in a patient with primary tuberculosis, disseminated tuberculosis with resultant miliary spread to multiple organs, including the lungs, occurs (Fig. 1.20). Miliary tuberculosis was discussed in Chapter 1.

Reactivation tuberculosis is the most common manifestation of tuberculosis among adults worldwide. Indeed, in a patient with any chronic upper lobe infiltrate, tuberculosis is the most likely diagnosis. Cavitation only intensifies this suspicion. In countries where tuberculosis is relatively uncommon, however, such as the United States, primary tuberculosis commonly occurs in adults. Thus, tuberculosis may appear as a patchy infiltrate in any lobe or as mediastinal adenopathy, both of which are manifestations of primary tuberculosis

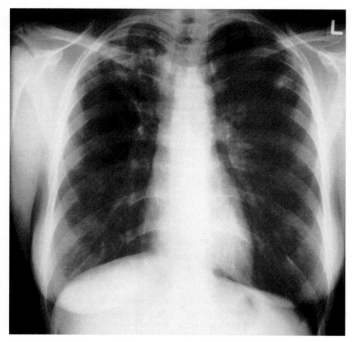

Figure 3.3. Reactivation tuberculosis. This 47-year-old man had a patchy infiltrate in the right upper lobe with cavitation, which is characteristic of tuberculosis.

Focal Alveolar Infiltrates

(Fig. 10.8). In addition, either primary or reactivation tuberculosis in adults may appear as a mass rather than an infiltrate, usually in an upper lobe.

Tuberculosis is spread by direct contact with people who have active disease. Thus, it is important to survey (by skin test, chest x-ray, or both) those who have had contact with patients having newly diagnosed tuberculosis. Drug therapy usually is effective in controlling this disease, though drug-resistant organisms are becoming more frequent, thereby making drug therapy more difficult.

Atypical Mycobacterial Infections

Runyon identified a number of mycobacterial organisms that he termed *atypical* or *nontuberculous mycobacteria*. For many years, these organisms were not thought to be pathogenic to humans. Subsequently, however, it has been recognized that most nontuberculous mycobacteria occasionally can be pathogenic and that several, such as *Mycobacterium avium-intracellulare* and *M. kansasii*, are fairly common pathogens in humans.

Unlike *M. tuberculosis*, atypical mycobacteria do not have a primary and a reactivation phase. All atypical mycobacteria represent primary infection and are spread by inhaling organisms found in water and soil. They are not spread by human contact. This is an important consideration, because unlike patients infected with *M. tuberculosis*, those infected with atypical mycobacteria are not infectious to others with whom they come in contact.

Radiographically, many of the infections caused by nontuberculous mycobacteria cannot be distinguished from infection with *M. tuberculosis*. They cause patchy upper lobe infiltrates, many of which are cavitary. These cavities often are thin-walled as well, which is considered to be a characteristic of *M. kansasii*.

Nontuberculous mycobacteria, however, also may cause several different patterns in the lung. These include patchy infiltrates in the middle or either lower lobe and frequently bronchiectasis in both lungs with patchy nodular infiltrates or cystic areas in both lung fields (Figs. 2.5 and 3.4).

These organisms usually are difficult to treat with drugs. They require prolonged therapy with multiple drugs.

Certain atypical mycobacteria occur with increased frequency in certain diseases. Thus, *M. fortuitum* occurs with some frequency in patients with achalasia, and *M. chelonei* occurs in patients with cystic fibrosis. *M. avium-intracellulare* is a very common pathogen in patients with AIDS but generally takes a different pattern in those patients with mediastinal adenopathy as the primary presentation.

Fungal Infections

Various fungi may cause alveolar pulmonary infiltrates. These include *Aspergillus* sp., *Blastomyces dermatitidis*, *Histoplasma capsulatum*, *Coccidioides immitis*, and *Cryptococcus neoformans*. All of these fungal infections can occur in patients with immunocompromise, particularly patients with AIDS.

Aspergillus Sp. Aspergillosis is one of the more interesting fungal infections because of the many ways that it can involve the lung. It may cause a chronic cavity, usually in an upper lobe, with an intracavitary mass (i.e., fungus ball) or mycetoma (Fig. 3.5). A mycetoma may be a manifestation of noninvasive or semi-invasive aspergillosis. In noninvasive aspergillosis, the organism inhabits a preexisting cavity within the lung. In semi-invasive aspergillosis, the organ-

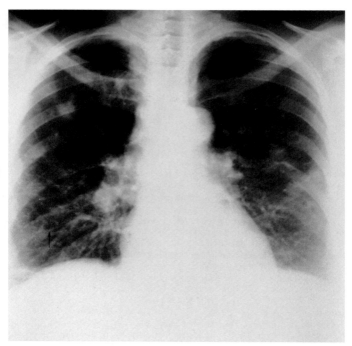

Figure 3.4. Infection with *Mycobacterium avium-intracellulare*. This 57-year-old man had patchy nodules throughout both lung fields, at least one of which was filled with air (*arrow*). These changes represent bronchiectasis and are a fairly characteristic finding in pulmonary infection with atypical mycobacteria in the normal host.

ism starts as a patchy infiltrate in an upper lobe and gradually develops a crescent as the infiltrate cavitates and finally emerges as a thick-walled—and subsequently a thin-walled—cavity with an intracavitary mass (Fig. 3.5). Both noninvasive and semi-invasive aspergillosis characteristically affect patients with mild immune abnormalities, such as those with sarcoidosis, alcoholism, or previous radiation exposure.

Aspergillus sp. are ubiquitous organisms found in the lungs of many normal individuals. The organism usually is nonpathogenic, but in patients with severe immunosuppression, this usually noninvasive organism becomes invasive. It characteristically takes the form of one or several patchy infiltrates in the lung fields, and it sometimes takes the form of very extensive bilateral infiltrates. It frequently is somewhat nodular as well, because of infarction created by the angioinvasive organism. Invasive aspergillosis most commonly occurs in patients with leukemia whose white-blood-cell counts are at their nadir because of drug therapy. It also may be seen in other patients with immunocompromise, such as those with AIDS or after bone marrow transplantation.

Focal Alveolar Infiltrates

Blastomyces Dermatitidis. Blastomycosis is a chronic infection that can occur anywhere in the lungs. It usually involves one focal area, but it occasionally can be multifocal. It may invade the chest wall, be cavitary, or both.

Histoplama Capsulatum. Histoplasmosis results from exposure to Histoplasma capsulatum, frequently as in the form of bird or bat excrement. It characteristically causes pulmonary nodules, either single or multiple, but it also may cause patchy infiltrates, usually in an upper lobe as a chronic manifestation of histoplasmosis. Occasionally, these infiltrates may be cavitary.

Coccidioides Immitis. Coccidioidomycosis is a disease of the San Joaquin Valley and adjacent areas in the western United States. Patients have single or multiple patchy infiltrates in one or both lungs. These infiltrates often are cavitary as well. A solitary thin-walled cavity often is a chronic manifestation of coccidioidomycosis. Like histoplasmosis, this disease frequently is self-limited but can exhibit a chronic phase, either as a solitary thin-walled cavity or as single or multiple infiltrates or cavitary disease.

Cryptococcus Neoformans. Cryptococcosis usually causes nodular disease in the normal host, but it also may cause patchy alveolar infiltrates.

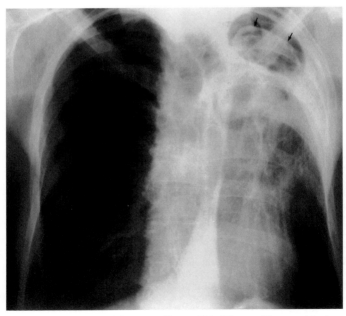

Figure 3.5. Left upper lobe aspergilloma. This 55-year-old man with alcoholism had a cavity in the left upper lobe with an intracavitary fungus ball (*arrows*). This is quite characteristic of noninvasive or semi-invasive aspergillosis.

Related Infections. Related infections can include those involving *Actinomyces* and *Nocardia* sp., which are bacterial organisms once thought to be fungi. These organisms cause chronic alveolar infiltrates in the lung or sometimes nodules. Actinomycosis may invade the chest wall and cause a pleural effusion. Infection with *Nocardia* sp. is seen in patients with pulmonary alveolar proteinosis and in those with immunosuppression.

Tumor

Tumor not uncommonly presents as solitary or multiple patchy alveolar infiltrates. Lymphoma is particularly likely to do this in young patients, and alveolar cell carcinoma presents in this fashion in older patients. Though not usually alveolar, metastatic carcinoma occasionally can present as an alveolar infiltrate.

Primary Carcinoma

Most primary carcinomas of the lung present as a poorly circumscribed nodule or an atelectasis. Primary lung carcinoma, however, sometimes will present as a solitary patchy alveolar infiltrate. This is especially true of the solitary-type bronchoalveolar carcinoma. Bronchoalveolar carcinoma also may present as multiple patchy nodules in one or both lungs (Fig. 3.6) or as a lobar infiltrate resembling lobar pneumonia, but this is a diffuse variant of bronchoalveolar carcinoma with a much worse prognosis than the solitary variant.

Lymphoma

Lymphoma fairly commonly causes patchy infiltrates in the lung (Fig. 3.7). In patients with Hodgkin's disease, this infiltrate is always accompanied or preceded by mediastinal adenopathy. Patients with non-Hodgkin's lymphoma may have pulmonary infiltrates without adenopathy. In all patients with lymphoma, these infiltrates may be cavitary as well.

Metastatic Carcinoma

Metastatic carcinoma usually is seen as single or multiple nodules or as diffuse lymphangitic tumor, but certain types may be alveolar. Choriocarcinoma characteristically causes alveolar metastasis when it metastasizes to the lung. Metastatic breast cancer usually causes pulmonary nodules or lymphangitic tumor when it spreads to the lung, and though not commonly alveolar, it is still the most common cause of alveolar metastases. In patients with breast carcinoma and a chronic infiltrate that resembles pneumonia, the diagnosis of metastatic tumor should be considered.

Pulmonary Infarction

Pulmonary embolism is a very common problem. Most patients with pulmonary emboli do not develop pulmonary infarction, however, because the dual blood supply to the lung prevents tissue infarction.

Pulmonary infarct appears radiographically as a wedge-shaped opacity in the lung field periphery. When large, the infarct will be segmental, and occasionally, pulmonary infarction may cause lobar consolidation, which cannot be distinguished from lobar pneumonia. Pulmonary infarction usually is accompanied by pleural effusion; thoracentesis often demonstrates a hemorrhagic effusion.

Focal Alveolar Infiltrates

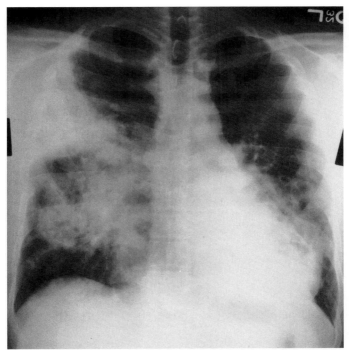

Figure 3.6. Bronchoalveolar carcinoma. Patchy infiltrates in both lower lobes and the right upper lobe are nonspecific but consistent with diffuse bronchoalveolar carcinoma.

The radiographic findings of pulmonary infarct are nonspecific and require confirmation by angiography, radionuclide scans, or computed tomography. Over time, a pulmonary infarct may be suspected on the basis of how the localized pulmonary infiltrate clears. Infarcts tend to "melt," changing from a wedge-shaped density to a rounded, peripheral density (i.e., Hampton's hump) and subsequently resulting in an area of focal pleural thickening. In addition, infarcts, unlike pneumonia, usually take many weeks to clear.

Radiation

Radiation causes an alveolar infiltrate in the area of the radiation portal. This portal has a well-defined margin; therefore, the radiation-induced change in the lung may be recognized by the sharply delineated edge of the infiltrate. Radiation consolidation occurs in the lung between 2 weeks and 1 year after the end of radiation therapy that includes part of the lung. When this infiltrate initially appears, it may be indistinguishable from pneumonia. As it progresses, however, it causes scarring and retraction of the lung, with a more dense area of con-

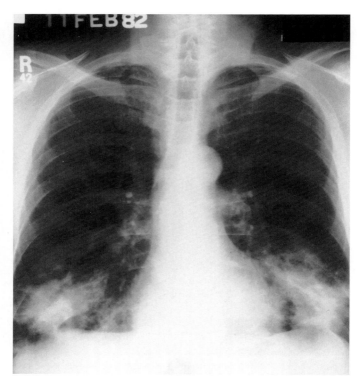

Figure 3.7. Pulmonary lymphoma. This 50-year-old man with cutaneous T-cell lymphoma (mycosis fungoides) had bilateral pulmonary infiltrates that proved to be pulmonary lymphoma at biopsy. Patients with Hodgkin's lymphoma almost always have associated adenopathy, whereas patients with non-Hodgkin's lymphoma may have pulmonary infiltrates as an isolated finding.

solidation. In the upper lobes, this frequently resembles pulmonary tuberculosis. In patients who underwent radiation therapy for primary lung carcinoma, it may be impossible to determine if residual tumor is present in the radiated area. Radiation-induced infiltrates sometimes are complicated by the superimposition of semi-invasive aspergillosis, with the formation of a mycetoma in the area of the radiation (Fig. 3.8).

Vasculitis

Some vasculitides involve the lung but only cause abnormalities in the appearance of the pulmonary vasculature. Others cause patchy infiltrates in the lungs. Primary among these latter vasculitides is Wegener's granulomatosis, which may present with a combination of chronic renal disease, sinus disease, and pulmonary infiltrates or nodules (Fig. 3.9). Only one of these three findings may occur, however, and limited pulmonary Wegener's granulomatosis is not unusual. Radiographically, Wegener's generally is seen as three or four patchy infiltrates, but it also may be solitary or have more numerous infiltrates. Occasionally, these infiltrates may be quite nodular as well, but they rarely are cavitary.

Other vasculitides can involve the lung in a similar fashion. Churg-Strauss vasculitis, which is a form of periarteritis nodosa with lung involvement, also may produce patchy alveolar infiltrates or present as nodules within the lungs. Lymphomatoid granulomatosis, which is a form of lymphoma with a vasculitis-like picture, also can involve the lung with single or multiple patchy alveolar nodules. Necrotizing sarcoid granulomatosis, which is a vasculitis-like presentation of sarcoid, causes patchy alveolar infiltrates as well.

Chronic Eosinophilic Pneumonia

Chronic eosinophilic pneumonia is an unusual disease of unknown origin that causes patchy alveolar infiltrates in the lungs. These infiltrates may be focal, but

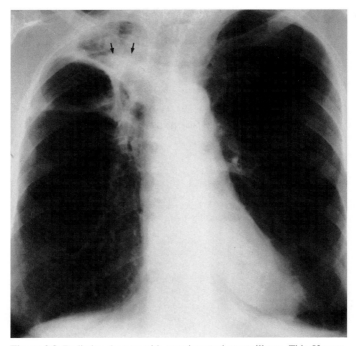

Figure 3.8. Radiation therapy with superimposed aspergilloma. This 52-year-old woman underwent radiation therapy of the right upper lobe for lung carcinoma and had a patchy infiltrate in the right upper lobe secondary to the radiation. She subsequently developed cavitation with a fungus ball (*arrows*), which is characteristic of noninvasive aspergillosis.

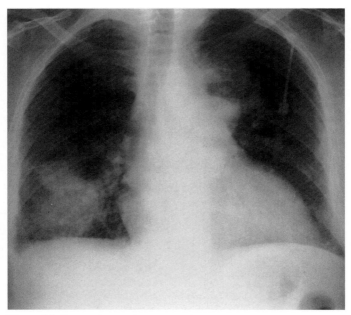

Figure 3.9. Wegener's granulomatosis. This 47-year-old man had patchy infiltrates in the right lower lobe and left upper lobe that proved to be Wegener's granulomatosis at biopsy.

they usually are bilateral and often are fairly symmetrical. Characteristically, they are peripheral and often predominantly involve the upper lung fields (Fig. 3.10). Occasionally, they may be cavitary. If untreated, they may progress to extensive pulmonary involvement and even death. This particular disease is exquisitely responsive to steroids and dramatically disappears after steroid therapy.

Acute eosinophilic pneumonia (i.e., Loeffler's syndrome) also may cause patchy alveolar infiltrates in both lungs. These infiltrates migrate from one area to another over a short period of time (days to weeks). It is usually a self-limited disease and may be caused by parasites or drugs, but it sometimes is idiopathic.

Other eosinophilic lung diseases such as allergic bronchopulmonary aspergillosis (ABPA) and Churg-Strauss (i.e., allergic vasculitis) also may cause patchy infiltrates in the lungs. ABPA more typically causes a bronchiectasis pattern.

Bronchiolitis Obliterans Organizing Pneumonia

Bronchiolitis obliterans organizing pneumonia is a lung reaction that is related to several other entities, but it often is idiopathic, having no association with another disease. It is seen particularly in patients with collagen vascular disease. It is very steroid-responsive and usually clears rapidly after their administration.

This type of pneumonia has several radiographic presentations. It frequently

Focal Alveolar Infiltrates

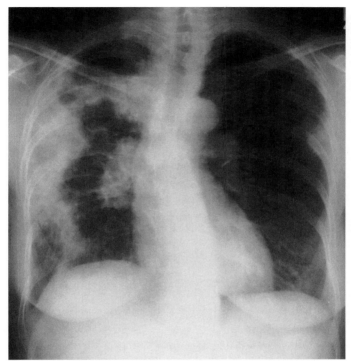

Figure 3.10. Chronic eosinophilic pneumonia. This 39-year-old woman with asthma had peripheral infiltrates in both lungs (though most markedly on the right side). Peripheral infiltrates are suggestive of chronic eosinophilic pneumonia as the diagnosis.

causes patchy alveolar infiltrates involving both lungs. Occasionally, however, it may cause a solitary alveolar infiltrate, or it may cause interstitial lung disease that is indistinguishable from idiopathic pulmonary fibrosis. It usually progresses slowly over time but may wax and wane, though this finding is unusual in patients with most lung diseases. Such waxing and waning (or improvement and then progression without any therapy) is suggestive of either bronchiolitis obliterans, organizing pneumonia, or vasculitis.

SUGGESTED READINGS

Albelda SM, Williams TM, Kern JA, Iozzo RV, Miller WT. Non-tuberculous mycobacterial infection in the acquired immunodeficiency syndrome: clinical, pathological and radiologic features. Radiology 1986;160:77–82.

Aronchick JM, Miller WT Jr. Disseminated nontuberculous mycobacterial infections in immunosuppressed patients. Semin Roentgenol 1993;28:150–157.

Churg A. Pulmonary angitis and granulomatosis revised. Hum Pathol 1983;14:868–883.

Conn DL. Pathogenic mechanisms in systemic vasculitis. Semin Respir Med 1989;10:122–125.

Genereux GP, Stillwell GA. The acute bacterial pneumonias. Semin Roentgenol 1980;15:9–16.

Greenspan RH. Ravin CR, Polansky SM, McLoud TC. Accuracy of the chest radiograph in the diagnosis of pulmonary embolism. Invest Radiol 1982;17:539–543.

James DG. Definition and classification of granulomatosis. Semin Respir Med 1986;8:1–9.

Miller WT, ed. Fungus diseases of the chest. Semin Roentgenol. Philadelphia: WB Saunders, Vol XXX1, l996.

Miller WT. Pulmonary infections. In: Taveras JM, Ferruci JT, eds. Radiology diagnosis—imaging intervention. Philadelphia: JB Lippincott, l988;1:1–29.

Miller WT, Husted J, Freiman D, Atkinson B, Pietra G. Bronchioloalveolar carcinoma: two clinical entities with one pathologic diagnosis. AJR 1978;130:905–912.

Miller WT, MacGregor RR. Tuberculosis: frequency of unusual radiographic findings. AJR 1978;130:867–875.

Miller WT Jr, Miller WT Sr. Pulmonary infections with atypical Mycobacteria in the normal host. Semin Roentgenol 1993;28:139–149.

Runyon LH. Anonymous mycobacteria in pulmonary disease. Med Clin North Am 1959;43:273–290.

Scanlon GT, Unber JD. The radiology of bacterial and viral pneumonias. Radiol Clin North Am l973;11:3l7–338.

Weisbrod Gl. Pulmonary angitis and granulomatosis: a review. J Can Assoc Radiol 1989;40:127–134.

Woodring JH. Pulmonary bacterial and viral infections. In: Freundlich, IM, Bragg, DG, eds. A radiologic approach to diseases of the chest. Baltimore: Williams & Wilkins, 1992:245–262.

4

Atelectasis

TYPES OF ATELECTASIS

Atelectasis can be divided into several different categories:

> 1. Passive.
> 2. Cicatricial.
> 3. Adhesive.
> 4. Resorption.

PASSIVE ATELECTASIS

Neuromuscular problems that interfere with the expansion of the chest wall or the diaphragm, such as paralysis of a hemidiaphragm, result in poor expansion of one or both lungs. Lack of expansion by the lung in this situation usually is not designated as *passive atelectasis*, though it could be.

Instead, we reserve the term for loss of volume or failure of expansion by the lung that occurs in a patient with an intrathoracic problem and that does not allow the lung to expand fully. If the patient has a pleural effusion or pneumothorax, the inherent elasticity of the lung causes the lung volume to be reduced (i.e., passive atelectasis) to the point at which intrathoracic pressure again is negative. With a very large pleural effusion or pneumothorax, the lung loses all of its elasticity—and consequently all of its volume. If the pleural effusion or pneumothorax then becomes still larger (i.e., tension physiology), the mediastinum shifts to the contralateral side.

In a similar fashion, a space-occupying lesion in the lung such as a large bulla or mass allows the adjacent lung to retract. Though sometimes termed *compressive atelectasis*, this really is a type of passive atelectasis.

Passive atelectasis is a common problem. In patients with chronic problems such as pleural effusion, passive atelectasis generally occurs to a greater degree in those areas where the effusion is larger. In an upright individual, this usually is in the lower lobes. In upright individuals with pneumothorax, however, air collects in the apices of the lungs, so the loss of volume is greater in the upper lung fields. Loss of volume in the area of a lung mass tends to be greater immediately adjacent to the lung mass or bulla.

COMMON CAUSES OF PASSIVE ATELECTASIS

Among the most common causes of passive atelectasis is atelectasis resulting from thoracic or abdominal pain. Patients with pain often alter their breathing pattern, thereby resulting in loss of volume in one or both lungs. This may involve the dependent portions of the lungs specifically and thus cause lobar atelectasis. Poor inspiration during the postoperative period probably is the most common cause of passive atelectasis.

Other common causes of passive atelectasis include:
1. Space-occupying lesion.
    A. Pleural effusion.
    B. Pneumothorax.
    C. Bullae.
    D. Ascites.
2. Neuromuscular disease.
    A. Diaphragmatic paralysis.
    B. Myasthenia gravis.
    C. Spinal cord injury.
    D. Stroke.

3. Thoracic or Abdominal Pain.
   A. Recent surgery.
   B. Trauma.
   C. Pulmonary embolism.
   D. Pleuritis.
   E. Inflammatory disease below the diaphragm.
      i. Pancreatitis.
      ii. Cholecystitis.
      iii. Peritonitis.
      iv. Subphrenic abscess.

Plate-like Atelectasis

Plate-like atelectasis is a special type of passive atelectasis in which the atelectasis occurs in a thin but wide fashion and resembles a plate or a line. This plate or line frequently parallels the diaphragm, but this type of atelectasis can occur in almost any direction (Fig. 4.1). It occurs most commonly in patients with poor diaphragmatic motion (e.g., individuals with obesity) or in patients with ascites, hepatomegaly, splenomegaly, or splinting of the diaphragm for some reason (often after surgery).

Cicatricial Atelectasis

Cicatricial atelectasis indicates the diffuse loss of volume that usually accompanies infiltrative processes of the lungs, such as those involved in most diffuse lung diseases. This type can occur with any interstitial lung disease, but certain diffuse lung diseases are much more marked by cicatricial atelectasis. Idiopathic pulmonary fibrosis and sarcoidosis are two processes that are accompanied by severe loss of volume.

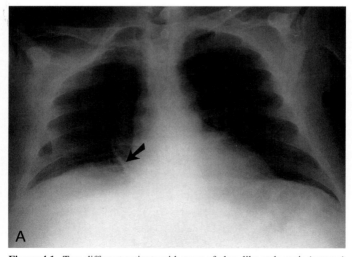

Figure 4.1. Two different patients with areas of plate-like atelectasis (*arrows*) on posteroanterior (**A**) and lateral (**B**) films.

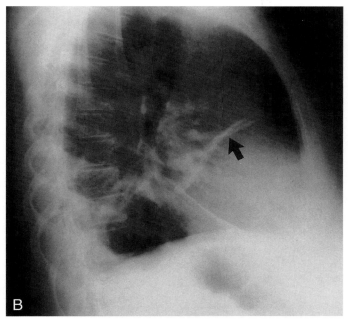

Figure 4.1. (*continued*)

Adhesive Atelectasis

Adhesive atelectasis, or microatelectasis, denotes alveolar collapse that occurs diffusely and often relates to abnormalities of surfactant. Surfactant deficiency syndrome or hyaline membrane disease in infants is a classic example of this type of atelectasis. In adults, this type may be seen in patients with adult respiratory distress syndrome and also is a prominent feature of radiation-induced changes that occur in the lung.

Resorption Atelectasis

The various types of atelectasis just described are important in explaining the appearance of the lung in differing situations. The overall term *atelectasis*, however, usually is associated with resorption atelectasis, which occurs when the bronchi are obstructed. This obstruction often results from blockage of a major airway, such as a lobar bronchus or main stem bronchus of one lung, but it also may result from blockage of multiple small bronchi in one lobe. This latter finding frequently occurs during the postoperative period or in critically ill patients.

The loss of volume necessary to indicate resorption atelectasis is quite variable. "Atelectasis" itself implies a loss of volume, but there may be no loss of volume in a patient with lobar obstruction. Two processes are present in the atelectatic lung. First, there is coaptation of the alveoli as the alveolar walls come together and the air is absorbed. If this is the only process, there may be 80% or

Atelectasis

90% loss of volume by the affected lobe. The second process, which also occurs in the obstructed lung, is filling of the alveoli with fluid. The lung ordinarily forms fluid in the obstructed lung, but if the fluid cannot escape, most of the atelectatic lung may fill with fluid and have very little coaptation of the alveoli. If this is the primary process, no loss of volume may occur in the lobe. Many might call this a "drowned lobe," but the process essentially is the same.

Lobar Atelectasis

Figure 4.2 shows atelectasis of the five lobes. Atelectasis may be minimal or very great depending on the amount of fluid remaining in the alveoli. Several principals should be remembered about lobar atelectasis:

1. All of the lobes are supplied by bronchi that begin at the hilum; therefore, all lobar atelectasis must point to the hilum.
2. An atelectatic lung always collapses medially.
3. The lower lobes collapse posteriorly, the left upper lobe anteriorly, and the right upper lobe and middle lobe concentrically.

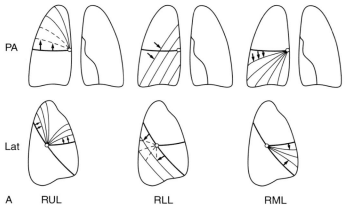

Figure 4.2. Atelectasis of the five lobes of the lung. The key to atelectasis is shifting of the fissures. This fissural shift may be minimal if the atelectasis is minimal and extensive if the atelectasis is severe. **A**. In right upper lobe atelectasis, the minor fissure moves up on the posteroanterior film, and the major and minor fissures move together on the lateral. In right lower lobe atelectasis, the major fissure becomes visible on the posteroanterior film and moves both down and medially; on the lateral film, the fissure moves posteriorly. A small part of the medial portion of the fissure extends upward to the hilum. In right middle lobe atelectasis, the minor fissure moves downward and medially on the posteroanterior film, and both fissures move together concentrically on the lateral film. **B**. In left upper lobe atelectasis, the major fissure moves anteriorly. On the posteroanterior film, this is seen as increased density over the left thorax, with loss of the cardiac border silhouette; on the lateral film, the major fissure moves anteriorly. A small part of the medial portion of the fissure extends down to the hilum, but this usually is not visible. In left lower lobe atelectasis, the major fissure becomes visible and moves both downward and medially on the posteroanterior film; the major fissure moves posteriorly on the lateral film.

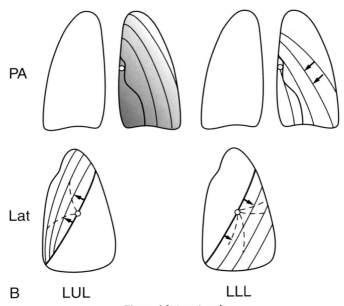

PA

Lat

B   LUL   LLL

Figure 4.2 (*continued*)

4. The major fissure is a plane and not a line. Therefore, in tight lower lobe atelectasis or left upper lobe atelectasis, the lateral portion of the fissure is far anterior (left upper lobe) or far posterior (lower lobe), but the medial portion of the fissure extends posterior (upper) or anterior (lower) to the level of the hilum. Only the lateral portion of the fissure may be visible, because it is tangential to the x-ray beam at imaging.

The major signs of an atelectatic lobe are consolidation of the involved lobe and displacement of the fissures, as described previously. Various secondary signs of atelectasis also are useful, however, particularly in very tight atelectasis. These secondary signs may indicate an abnormal chest film and lead one to search for an atelectatic lobe that may not be immediately obvious. Such secondary signs include:

1. Hyperinflation of the remaining lobes on the ipsilateral side.
2. Stretching of the vessels on the ipsilateral side.
3. Hilar changes.
   A. Displacement: The hilum is displaced upward in upper lobe atelectasis and downward in lower lobe atelectasis.
   B. Size: The hilum appears to be smaller in the ipsilateral lung, because the vessels in the atelectatic lobe that ordinarily comprise a portion of the hilum no longer can be seen. (They are silhouetted out by the atelectatic lobe.)
4. Shift of various anatomic structures.
   A. The mediastinum may be shifted to the ipsilateral side.
   B. The ipsilateral diaphragm may be elevated.

    C.   The chest wall may be reduced in size on the ipsilateral side, with the ribs being closer together on that side.
  5. Juxtaphrenic peak.

Decreased volume of the hemithorax produces traction on the diaphragm at the site of the inferior pulmonary ligament. This is termed the *juxtaphrenic peak*.

Lobar atelectasis may be mimicked by lobectomy. After lobectomy, the characteristic secondary signs of lobar atelectasis should be present, and occasionally, a density can be seen in the area of the above-mentioned lobectomy that resembles an atelectatic lung. This density is caused by pleural fluid or thickening at the site of the previous lobe or by a shift of the mediastinum, with mediastinal fat filling the space and simulating atelectasis of the surgically removed lobe. This is particularly true in a left upper lobectomy.

Lobar atelectasis is the usual finding in patients with resorption atelectasis, but more than one lobe may be involved. On the right side, the right middle and right lower lobe can be involved by an obstructive lesion in the intermediate bronchus. In addition, obstruction of the main stem bronchus can cause atelectasis of an entire lung on either side.

Segmental Atelectasis

Atelectasis of a segment is uncommon, because segmental obstruction usually is masked by collateral air drift between the alveoli of the obstructed segment and the alveoli of surrounding unobstructed segments. This keeps the obstructed segment aerated, and atelectasis does not occur. Such collateral air drift occurs through interalveolar communications (i.e., the pores of Kohn and canals of Lambert).

Nonetheless, one sometimes may encounter segmental atelectasis. Segmental atelectasis usually occurs in patients with long-standing segmental obstruction, and it frequently indicates a low-grade tumor such as a carcinoid, a benign tumor such as a hamartoma, or an inflammatory process. Higher-grade malignancies usually do not cause segmental atelectasis and first become visible through lobar obstruction.

CAUSES OF RESORPTION ATELECTASIS

Causes of resorption atelectasis include:

> 1. Postoperative atelectasis, or atelectasis in a critically ill patient.
> 2. Carcinoma of the lung.
> 3. Metastatic tumor.
> 4. Bronchial adenomas.
> 5. Inflammatory causes.
>   A. Right middle lobe syndrome.
>   B. Plasma cell granuloma.
> 6. Foreign body.

Posoperative Atelectasis

In postoperative patients as well as in others with thoracic or abdominal pain, generalized passive atelectasis results from poor diaphragmatic motion. Lobar atelectasis also is very common, particularly in the lower lobes (the left more common than the right). Similarly, in critically ill patients, particularly those in the intensive care unit or with abdominal pain and splinting of one or both diaphragms, lobar atelectasis is very common (Fig. 4.3). Like postoperative atelectasis, this type usually involves the lower lobe.

These patients may have moderate loss of volume by the involved atelectatic lobe, but this loss of volume often is only minimal. An air bronchogram is fairly common in these patients, though it also may be absent. Atelectasis usually involves the entire lobe, but in the lower lobe, it may spare the superior segment and affect only the basal segments of the lower lobe.

The atelectasis in these patients may result from obstruction of the lobar bronchus by a mucous plug or aspiration. Usually, however, the main stem bronchus is not obstructed, and the obstruction actually involves multiple small bronchi throughout the involved lobe.

Because there is little loss of volume and frequently an air bronchogram, this type of atelectasis cannot be distinguished radiographically from pneumonia. Therefore, the distinction must be made on the basis of clinical grounds. Generally, in postoperative or critically ill patients with lower lobe consolidation, atelectasis is a more likely cause of this consolidation.

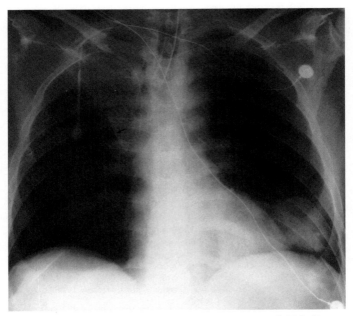

Figure 4.3. Right upper lobe atelectasis in the intensive care unit. This 47-year-old man with metastatic tumor (note the left lower lobe nodule) had right upper lobe atelectasis with an elevated minor fissure (*arrows*). Atelectasis of various lobes is common in the intensive care setting and in postoperative patients. Lower lobe atelectasis is the most common and is most frequently seen in these settings.

Atelectasis

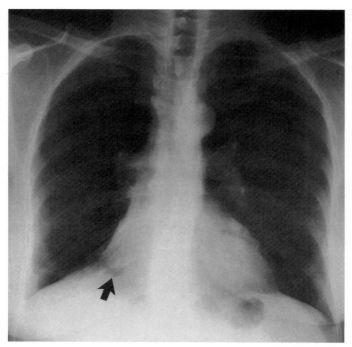

Figure 4.4. Right lower lobe atelectasis caused by lung carcinoma. This 60-year-old woman had tight atelectasis of the right lower lobe. The medial portion of the right hemidiaphragm is indistinct (*arrow*), but the secondary signs of atelectasis include a small right hemithorax, small pulmonary vessels on the right, and a small hilum. The lateral film (not shown) was unremarkable.

Carcinoma of the Lung

Bronchogenic carcinoma can present in several fashions: a solitary pulmonary nodule of various size, a patchy pulmonary infiltrate, mediastinal adenopathy with no obvious pulmonary lesion, and multifocal alveolar nodules (i.e., bronchoalveolar carcinoma). One of the more common presentations of bronchogenic carcinoma, however, is a central lesion (Figs. 4.4 and 4.5) that obstructs a large airway, usually a lobar bronchus but sometimes the intermediate

Figure 4.5. Left upper lobe atelectasis secondary to lung carcinoma. Posteroanterior (**A**) and lateral (**B**) films show atelectasis of the left upper lobe without loss of volume. The heart border is obscured by the atelectasis, and the major fissure (*arrows*) on the lateral film (**B**) is minimally displaced. In another patient, posteroanterior (**C**) and lateral (**D**) films show very tight atelectasis of the left upper lobe. The left lung is totally collapsed around the left hilum (**C**; *arrows*), and the major fissure (*arrows*) is displaced far anteriorly (**D**).

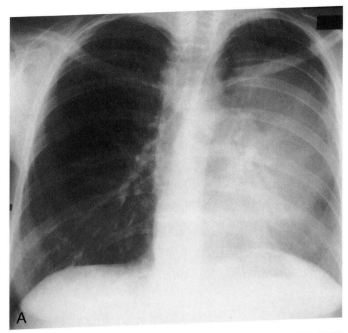

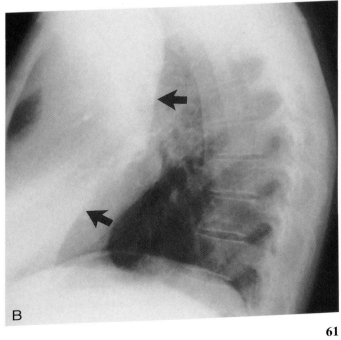

61

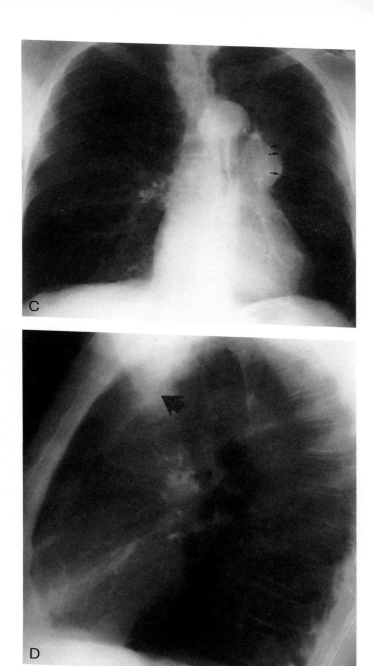

Figure 4.5. (*continued*)

bronchus or entire lung. This causes lobar atelectasis and is the most common cause of this type of atelectasis among nonhospitalized patients.

The degree of atelectasis of the lobe varies from minimal to very severe. There frequently is mediastinal and hilar adenopathy accompanying the atelectatic lobe, and there is almost never an air bronchogram in this type of obstructive atelectasis. In patients who present with these findings, bronchogenic carcinoma is a highly likely diagnosis. Endoscopy is indicated to identify the tumor and to exclude other causes of lobar atelectasis.

Metastatic Tumor

A metastatic tumor usually is not endobronchial. It generally goes to the lung periphery, where the capillaries are much more numerous and the metastases tend to lodge. A few tumors tend to metastasize to lobar bronchi, however, and may present with atelectasis (Fig. 4.6). As usual, breast carcinoma is the most common tumor to do this. Melanoma and lymphoma are other tumors that metastasize to the bronchi with some frequency, and any tumor can do it on occasion. Lymph nodes in the mediastinum or hilum can compress the bronchi but

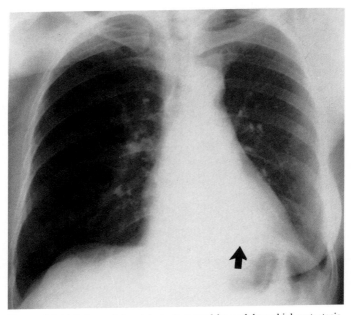

Figure 4.6. Left lower lobe atelectasis caused by endobronchial metastasis. This 43-year-old woman had an absent right breast. The medial side of the left hemidiaphragm cannot be identified (*arrow*), because of left lower lobe consolidation (silhouette sign). No vessels can be seen through the heart, because the left lower lobe is densely consolidated. Secondary signs of atelectasis include a small hemithorax and an inferiorly displaced left hilum. The lateral film was unremarkable and is not shown.

almost never cause lobar atelectasis. If atelectasis is present, an endobronchial tumor usually is present; this is an important consideration in patients with lymphoma.

Bronchial Adenomas

A group of low-grade lung carcinomas have been erroneously termed *bronchial adenoma*, which is a name that would imply a benign diagnosis. These are not benign tumors, however. They are low-grade malignancies. Among these, in order of frequency, are carcinoid, adenocystic carcinoma or cylindroma, and mucoepidermoid carcinoma.

Carcinoid tumor occurs in relatively young patients (in their thirties and forties). It most commonly is central (in the area of the hilum) but may be a peripheral nodule. It often causes lobar atelectasis (Fig. 4.7). Segmental atelecta-

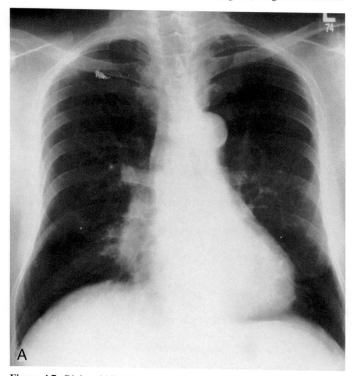

Figure 4.7. Right middle lobe atelectasis caused by endobronchial carcinoid. This 35-year-old woman had tight right middle lobe atelectasis. The heart border is blurred out (silhouette sign) on the posteroanterior film (**A**), and the major and minor fissures (arrows) are displaced on the lateral film (**B**). This tight right middle lobe atelectasis resulted from a carcinoid tumor of the right middle lobe bronchus.

Atelectasis

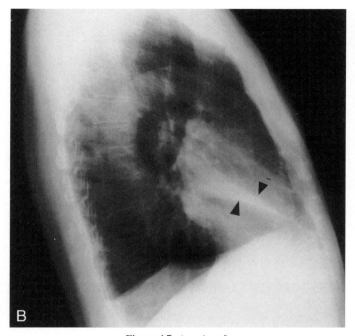

Figure 4.7. (*continued*)

sis is a relatively rare finding, but carcinoid tumor is very high on the list of endobronchial lesions that cause segmental atelectasis. Bronchial carcinoids are extremely vascular tumors and often cause hemoptysis. Considering this vascularity, most endoscopists will not biopsy a "cherry red" lesion that is suggestive of a carcinoid tumor, because a biopsy may lead to excessive bleeding. In most cases, surgeons proceed directly to surgery without a diagnosis established on the basis of biopsy findings. Because this tumor frequently is central, innovative types of bronchial resection and anastomoses often are necessary to preserve as much lung as possible.

Cylindromas usually are central lesions that involve the trachea and tracheal bifurcation, but occasionally, they can involve the hilum and present as a hilar lesion. They are almost never a solitary nodule in the lung periphery. Mucoepidermoid carcinomas usually are hilar and are the bronchial adenoma most likely to cause hilar and mediastinal adenopathy.

Inflammatory Causes

Most chronic infections of the lung cause patchy infiltrates. Rarely, however, tuberculosis in particular and fungus disease on occasion may present as lobar atelectasis when they produce an endobronchial mass that obstructs the bronchus. Most inflammatory causes of lobar atelectasis are nonspecific infec-

Atelectasis

tions of a lobe, which often are recurrent and lead to chronic bronchiectasis and loss of volume by the involved lobe.

Right Middle Lobe Syndrome

Right middle lobe syndrome is most common in the right middle lobe, but it can occur in any lobe. If the middle lobe is involved, this is called the right middle lobe syndrome (see Fig. 2.4). These patients frequently suffer from atelectasis of the involved lobe for many years. Bronchoscopy is indicated at least once during the disease to be certain the atelectasis is not caused by a lung carcinoma or by a low-grade endobronchial tumor (e.g., a carcinoid). In most cases, these patients are relatively asymptomatic, but they may require antibiotics for treatment of repeated episodes of infection.

It once was thought that right middle lobe syndrome was caused by enlarged lymph nodes obstructing the bronchus. Bronchoscopists have shown that bronchi in patients with right middle lobe syndrome are patent, however. The atelectasis results from obstruction of smaller bronchi. Patients with right middle lobe syndrome frequently have enlarged hilar lymph nodes, probably because of the chronic inflammation, but as mentioned, lymph nodes almost never cause bronchial obstruction by external compression.

Sarcoid is another inflammatory lesion that commonly causes endoscopically visible endobronchial masses. It seldom causes lobar atelectasis, however.

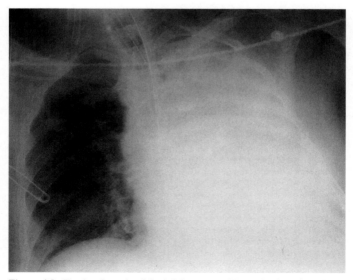

Figure 4.8. Total atelectasis of the left lung caused by aspiration of a chicken bone. This 60-year-old man had a previous history of lung carcinoma, and atelectasis of the left lung was thought to be the result of recurrent tumor. Bronchoscopy revealed a chicken bone, however, the removal of which relieved the obstruction of the left main stem bronchus.

Plasma Cell Granuloma

Another unusual endobronchial inflammatory lesion that may cause atelectasis is endobronchial plasma cell granuloma (i.e., inflammatory pseudotumor). This is more common among children than adults but still occurs in both groups. Plasma cell granuloma also may present as a solitary nodule in the lung. This nodule is a collection of plasma cells and is thought to be postinflammatory in origin.

Foreign Body

Foreign body of the bronchus is relatively uncommon in adults (Fig. 4.8). It sometimes is seen after use of an anesthetic, however, when the patient inhales some foreign object (occasionally a portion of his or her dentures). Foreign bodies are much more common in children, and they are a particularly difficult problem if they are vegetable material (e.g., a peanut), which tends to expand and swell in the bronchus and may be difficult to remove.

Endobronchial hamartoma is a rare cause of atelectasis. Most hamartomas are peripheral nodules.

SUGGESTED READINGS

Bramen SS, Whitcomb ME. Endobronchial metastases. Arch Intern Med 1975;135:543–547.

Lubert M, Krause GR. Patterns of lobar collapse as observed radiographically. Radiology 1951;56:165–182.

Pare JAP, Fraser RG. Atelectasis. In: Synopsis of diseases of the chest. Philadelphia: WB Saunders, 1983:169–188.

Proto AV, Tocino I. Radiographic manifestations of lobar collapse. Semin Roentgenol 1980;15:117–173.

Pugatch RD, Schaffer K. Primary pulmonary neoplasm. In: Freundlich IM, Bragg DG, eds. A radiologic approach to diseases of the chest. Baltimore: Williams & Wilkins, 1992:321–336.

Sutnick AJ, Soloff LA. Atelectasis with pneumonia: a pathophysiologic study. Ann Intern Med 1964;60:39–46.

Solitary Pulmonary Nodule **5**

DIFFERENTIATING NODULAR DENSITIES

A pulmonary nodule is a well-circumscribed (or fairly well-circumscribed) nodular density in any part of the lung. The nodule is considered to be solitary if the film shows only one. Often, however, a computed tomographic (CT) scan shows that multiple nodules actually are present, which immediately changes the diagnostic possibilities.

It is important to be certain that a true pulmonary nodule is present and the density depicted is not some overlying structure. **Overlying structures that commonly mimic pulmonary nodules include the nipple shadow; a rib fracture, bone island, or other nodular density in the rib; a skin nodule caused by a wart, mole, neurofibroma, and so on; and a combination of normal vascular and bony structures creating the false perception of a nodule.**

Nipple Shadows, Warts, and Cutaneous Nodules

Nipple shadows, warts, or other cutaneous nodules that project into the air from the chest wall may create a nodular density identical to that of a lung nodule surrounded by air in the alveoli. The nipple probably is the most common problem culprit. Paradoxically, the nipple shadow is more likely to create an apparent lung nodule in male than in female patients. The male nipple shadow is more likely to overlie the lung, whereas the female nipple shadow frequently overlies the upper abdomen and is not an imaging problem. The nipple is easily identified by routine use of nipple markers during all outpatient examinations. Small opaque markers also can be used to identify other cutaneous nodules when such densities likely are the cause of perceived pulmonary nodules.

Rib Fracture

Healing rib fractures may resemble a pulmonary nodule and be mistaken for one. Similarly, a bone island in the rib also may be perceived as a pulmonary nodule. A bone island is a small, round area of sclerotic bone; this is a normal variation in the ribs of some patients.

Bony and Vascular Shadows

The most common cause of perceived nodules probably is a combination of bony and vascular shadows. Experienced radiologists usually can distinguish true from false nodules, but even in their hands, a certain number of repeat examinations are necessary to show that a concatenation of vascular and bony shadows is indeed that and not a true pulmonary nodule. In our department, repeat imaging for what proves to be a normal finding are performed in 3% to 5% of outpatient examinations. (We routinely use nipple markers as well, so the nipple is seldom a problem.)

DETECTING A PULMONARY NODULE

If one is uncertain regarding a possible pulmonary nodule on a chest film, repeat examination rather than CT is indicated. This repeat examination should include the projection that showed the perceived nodule (usually the posteroanterior but sometimes the lateral film) as well as oblique films. Oblique films alone are not sufficient, however. A repeat film similar to the original projection is needed to be absolutely certain if a perceived nodule is actually present, because a true nodule may be poorly perceived on oblique films.

Solitary Pulmonary Nodule

If one is absolutely certain that a nodular density is present, CT should be performed to determine if multiple pulmonary nodules are present. Before CT, however, it is wise to wait 7 to 10 days and then repeat the original examination. Many perceived nodules are actually inflammatory nodules and will become smaller or even disappear completely during that time. Thus, the more expensive CT can be avoided, and the brief delay required by this process should have no significant effect if the nodule is malignant.

A pulmonary nodule often is seen in retrospect, having been missed at the time of the initial examination. The radiologist is constantly searching for pulmonary nodules, but such a nodule fairly frequently is overlooked. In the 1990s, for example, two different studies were designed to detect cancer in cigarette smokers through screening films taken at 4- to 6-month intervals. The results of these studies showed that, in retrospect, lung cancers were detectable 90% (Mayo Clinic study) and 60% (Memorial Hospital study) of the time on one or more films taken 4 months to several years before the cancer was actually diagnosed. Thus, even expert radiologists who double-read these films and specifically looked for signs of cancer overlooked those early signs, many of which were pulmonary nodules.

The size of a detectable nodule varies with its location in the lung. If a nodule is very peripheral, one as small as 3 mm in diameter may be detected, particularly when an older film does not show it. Nodules of several centimeters may be overlooked, however, when they are adjacent to the hilum, where the confusing shadows of the large vessels are present.

The most useful tool in understanding the nature of a solitary pulmonary nodule is a previous film. Frequently, such a film shows that the pulmonary nodule either was or was not there, and it also can provide an idea of the rapidity of growth. If the nodule was not depicted 4 to 6 weeks previously and now is of moderate size, it likely is an inflammatory nodule. If the nodule was depicted 1 or more years ago and has not changed, it almost certainly is benign (probably a granuloma). If the nodule is growing very slowly, it probably is a hamartoma, but slow growth also can occur in low-malignancy nodules (e.g., carcinoid tumor).

CAUSES

Common causes of a solitary pulmonary nodule include:

1. Malignancy.
   A. Primary.
   B. Metastatic.
   C. Lymphoma.
   D. Benign.
2. Tumor-like conditions.
   A. Inflammatory pseudotumors.
   B. Amyloidosis.
3. Infection.
   A. Pneumonia.
   B. Granuloma.
4. Pulmonary infarct.
5. Arteriovenous malformation.
6. Mucoid impaction.

7. Conglomerate mass of silicosis.
8. Necrobiotic nodule.
9. Developmental anomalies.
   A. Bronchogenic cyst.
   B. Pulmonary sequestration.
   C. Cystic adenomatoid malformation.

Malignancy

Primary

Primary carcinoma of the lung is a very common pulmonary nodule. It probably is the most important one as well, because early detection and removal can be life-saving. In some patients, the radiographic characteristics of the nodules are strongly suggestive of a primary carcinoma. If the chest film or CT scan shows a spiculated border to the lesion (Fig. 5.1), associated hilar and mediastinal adenopathy, or evidence of metastases to other structures (e.g., bones, liver, adrenals), the diagnosis of primary lung carcinoma can be strongly suspected.

In many other patients, however, there are no specific radiographic findings. A lung carcinoma can be quite smooth or very irregular. It can be cavitary, and it may contain a small amount of calcification. It can be of almost any size, from

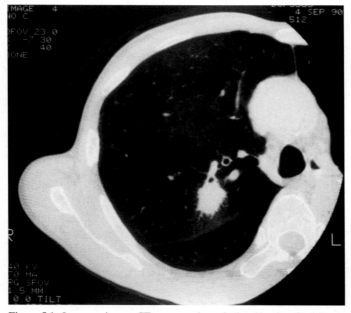

Figure 5.1. Lung carcinoma. CT scan reveals a spiculated border of a right upper lobe nodule. This is characteristic of a primary lung carcinoma and sometimes may be seen on the plain film.

Solitary Pulmonary Nodule

very small or very large, and it can occur at almost any age (particularly in those older than 30 years). Thus, a primary lung carcinoma must always be suspected in patients with a solitary nodule having no characteristics to indicate a definitely benign lesion.

Metastatic

It is not unusual for metastatic tumor to present as a solitary nodule in the lung. This is fairly common with metastases from the breast, kidney, and colon. It also is fairly common with melanoma and various soft-tissue and bone sarcomas. These are only some of the more common instances, however. A solitary metastasis can happen with any malignancy.

It is very common for the chest film to show a solitary nodule but for the CT scan to show several nodules. Multiple pulmonary nodules increases the likelihood of metastatic disease as a cause.

In addition, primary lung carcinoma commonly is associated with some other malignancy. Thus, patients with a known extrathoracic primary malignancy may have CT scans that show a solitary pulmonary nodule with the characteristics of a primary lung tumor. If the solitary nodule is spiculated and not smooth, the diagnosis of a metastatic tumor is not likely. Similarly, if ipsilateral hilar and mediastinal node metastases are present, the diagnosis of a primary lung carcinoma is strongly favored. Certain remote tumors, however, also may metastasize to the mediastinal lymph nodes as well as to the lung; these include breast, kidney, and testicular tumors as well as melanoma.

In patients with a known primary tumor and a solitary lung nodule, further workup is necessary to determine the nature of the nodule. This usually means fine-needle or thoracoscopic biopsy.

Lymphoma

Lymphoma may present as multiple pulmonary nodules, but it rarely presents as a solitary pulmonary nodule. The exception is lymphoma that involves bronchus-associated lymphoid tissue (BALT). This type of lymphoma usually presents as a solitary nodule but is a localized, low-grade malignancy. Cure is usually achieved by surgery.

Benign

Hamartoma is the most common benign tumor involving the lung. It also is the most common benign tumor to be seen as a solitary pulmonary nodule. It can be of any size, from several millimeters to as larger as 10 cm. It may contain characteristic "popcorn" calcification (Fig. 5.2) or have visible fat within as depicted on plain films or CT scans. If older films are available, the growth rate of this tumor is seen to be very slow.

Hamartomas once were thought to be developmental malformations. Today, however, most histopathologists now believe they are a true benign tumor. Other benign tumors (e.g., chondroma) also occasionally may occur in the lung.

Tumor-Like Conditions

Inflammatory Pseudotumors

An uncommon cause of pulmonary nodules is a group of conditions termed *inflammatory pseudotumors*. These include plasma cell granuloma, histiocytoma,

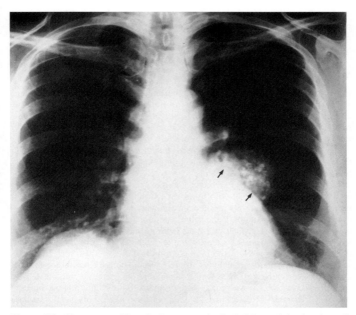

Figure 5.2. Hamartoma. Note the large mass in the left lower lobe, just lateral to the left heart border (*arrows*). Multiple areas of calcification (popcorn calcification) are characteristic of a hamartoma.

and pseudolymphoma. Plasma cell granuloma is more common among children. It usually causes a solitary pulmonary nodule, it also may present (in children or adults) as an endobronchial lesion. Histiocytoma usually presents as a solitary nodule. Pseudolymphoma can be a tumor-like condition and present as a solitary nodule, but it more commonly occurs as multiple nodules and may be a precursor of lymphoma or be confused with true lymphoma.

Amyloidosis

Another tumor-like condition that can present as a solitary pulmonary nodule is amyloidosis. Amyloidosis is rare, however, and usually presents as multiple pulmonary nodules.

Intrapulmonary lymph node is another condition that may create a solitary nodule. The diagnosis usually cannot be established short of surgical removal. If older films are available, this usually is seen to be a stable lesion.

Infection

Pneumonia

Pneumonia is an important cause of solitary pulmonary nodules. Pneumonia sometimes is very nodular in shape during its acute presentation (i.e., round

Solitary Pulmonary Nodule

pneumonia). In other cases, as pneumonia clears, it organizes into an amorphous mass (i.e., organizing pneumonia) (Fig. 5.3). Because of these two possibilities, delayed films should be obtained 1 to 2 weeks after the initial film before proceeding with the workup of a pulmonary nodule. Round pneumonia usually clears fairly rapidly, but organizing pneumonia may take many months to clear. As long as the nodule is getting smaller, however, an inflammatory process is strongly favored.

Granuloma

A granuloma secondary to previous primary tuberculosis or to a fungal infection (e.g., histoplasmosis, coccidioidomycosis) is the most common benign pulmonary nodule. In some patients, the characteristic calcification—central calcification, bulls-eye calcification, or popcorn calcification (Fig. 5.4)—may be present in the nodule. These are clear indications of a benign nodule. Though likely to indicate a granuloma, eccentric calcification can sometimes be seen in tumors growing around a preexisting granulomatous calcification. Thus, a nodule with eccentric calcification merits follow-up. CT numbers (Hounsfield units [HU]) can be used indicate calcification within the tumor, and a special phan-

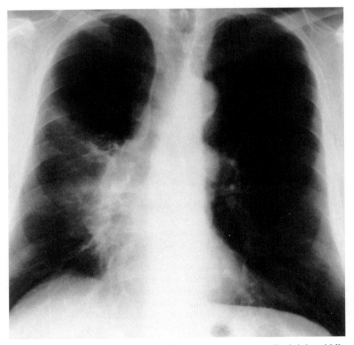

Figure 5.3. Organizing pneumonia. A large, poorly circumscribed right middle lobe mass in this 60-year-old man was unchanging. At surgery, this mass proved to be organizing pneumonia.

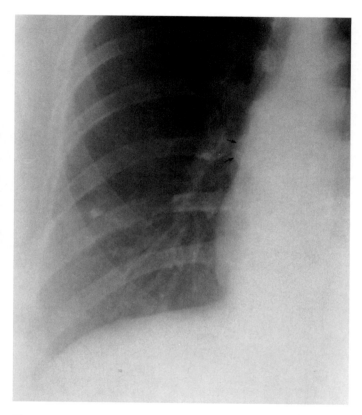

Figure 5.4. Right lower lobe granuloma. The densely calcified nodule in the right lower lobe is a granuloma from previous histoplasmosis or tuberculosis. Note also the calcified mediastinal lymph nodes (*arrows*).

tom has been constructed to measure the HU of the pulmonary nodule against a phantom reconstructed to simulate the pulmonary nodule. This way, the density of the pulmonary nodule can be measured accurately, even if one CT scanner is calibrated quite differently from another.

In our experience, measuring the HU of pulmonary nodules has not been very useful. When such measurements are positive, calcification is quite obvious on the plain films or thin-section CT scans. When such measurements are indeterminate, no calcification is seen, and the HU thus is not helpful.

Again, older films are useful for establishing the benign nature of a granuloma. If an older film shows that the nodule has not grown for 1 year or longer, the nodule probably is a granuloma. If the older film shows the nodule has grown very slowly in that time, it probably is a hamartoma or some other benign tumor. Certain malignant tumors such as carcinoid or solitary bron-

Solitary Pulmonary Nodule

choalveolar carcinoma also grow slowly, however, but at a faster rate than hamartomas.

Pulmonary Infarct

Pulmonary infarcts occasionally can present as a pulmonary nodule. The infarct usually is recognized in a patient with the symptoms of pulmonary embolism. If the embolism is not recognized, however, the patient may present with a solitary nodule, which is actually a pulmonary infarct. Pulmonary infarcts usually are peripheral and tend to have a wider diameter against the pleura than they do centrally. On follow-up films, they tend to become progressively more peripheral or to "melt" as the infarct ages. There often is significant pleural scarring associated with the infarct. Dog heartworm is a rare infestation in humans that also can cause pulmonary infarction and present as a pulmonary nodule.

Most pulmonary nodules do not have a shape that indicates a specific diagnosis. Arteriovenous malformation and mucoid impaction of the bronchus, however, usually have a characteristic radiographic appearance that is suggestive of the correct diagnosis.

Arteriovenous Malformation

In arteriovenous malformation (AVM), the supplying artery usually is slightly larger than the other arteries in the nearby lung, and the nodule results from dilatation of the distal end of the pulmonary vein that is involved in the AVM. As the vein proceeds toward the pulmonary hilum, it is dilated and serpiginous. The characteristic shape of an AVM is a nodule with a serpiginous tail, and it often is seen on the chest film. If it is recognized, no further workup is required (Fig. 5.5). If it is not recognized on the chest film, it may be seen on a CT scan. If it is suspected but not definitely diagnosed, enhancement of the AVM can be shown on either CT scans or magnetic resonance (MR) images. An arteriogram usually is not necessary to establish the diagnosis, but most AVMs should be embolized because of the high incidence of associated brain abscess. Thus, a diagnostic and a therapeutic procedure can be performed simultaneously. If AVMs are extensive, they may cause hypoxia because of arteriovenous shunting of unoxygenated blood; this is another indication for embolization.

Mucoid Impaction

A second lesion that may be quite characteristic on the plain film is mucoid impaction of the bronchus (Fig. 5.6). This lesion is recognized by the branching appearance of the nodule. Multiple branches or a nodule that appears to be have horns, which represent branching structures, may be seen. This characteristic appearance allows the nodule to be identified as mucoid impaction, but it does not indicate the cause of the impaction. Mucoid impaction of the bronchus is a characteristic finding with allergic bronchopulmonary aspergillosis. Allergic bronchopulmonary aspergillosis usually is a multifocal disease and is less likely to present as a solitary nodule, though it may do so on occasion. Other causes of solitary mucoid impaction include obstruction of the bronchus by a tumor, which often is benign (e.g., a carcinoid or hamartoma) but sometimes is lung carcinoma. Mucoid impaction of the bronchus also may result from inflammatory stenosis of the bronchus and has been seen in patients with tuberculosis and in those with atypical mycobacterial infections.

75

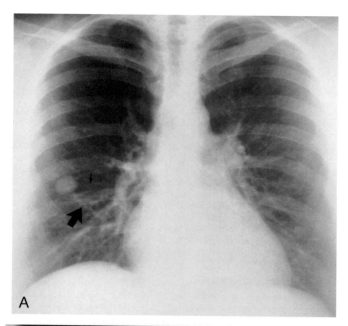

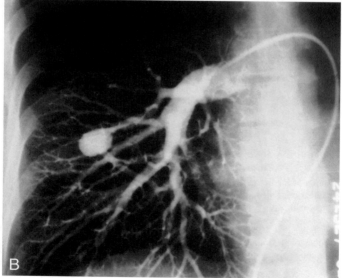

Figure 5.5. Arteriovenous malformation. AVM presents as a solitary nodule in the right midlung field. A feeding artery (*small arrow*) and draining vein (*large arrow*) can be identified on both the plain chest film (**A**) and the pulmonary arteriogram (**B**).

Solitary Pulmonary Nodule

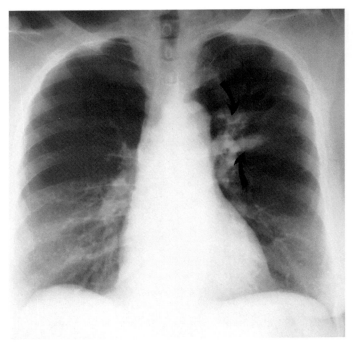

Figure 5.6. Mucoid impaction of the bronchus caused by allergic aspergillosis. Note the characteristic branching pattern of an obstructed bronchus in the left upper lobe (*arrows*) in this 34-year-old woman with asthma. This is characteristic of allergic bronchopulmonary aspergillosis, but it also can be seen with obstructive lesions of the bronchus secondary to tumor.

Conglomerate Mass of Silicosis

There are some conditions in which the patient's clinical history is suggestive of the diagnosis. In silicosis, a conglomerate mass may be seen as a solitary nodule in an upper lobe. Conglomerate masses often are bilateral (Fig. 5.7), and they usually are associated with evidence of silicosis elsewhere in the lung. In addition, the lung peripheral to the conglomerate mass frequently shows emphysematous change. Initially, the conglomerate mass appears to be an ill-defined density, but it subsequently organizes into a more sharply delimited mass that migrates toward the hilum as the bullae peripheral to the conglomerate mass enlarge. The diagnosis usually can be suspected on the basis of any individual film, but older films are extremely useful to see how the mass has developed. It may be difficult to differentiate a conglomerate mass from pulmonary tuberculosis or a primary lung tumor.

Solitary Pulmonary Nodule

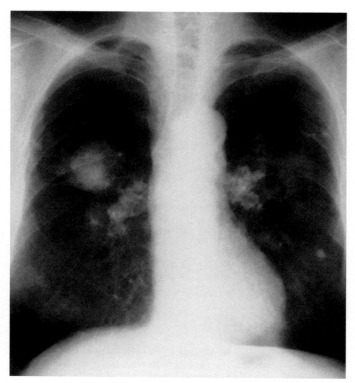

Figure 5.7. Conglomerate masses of silicosis. Mild interstitial disease is not very apparent in this 59-year-old coal miner. Note, however, the well-defined right upper lobe and the poorly defined left upper lobe nodule (*arrows*). These are typical of conglomerate masses of silicosis.

Necrobiotic Nodule

One mass that is suggested by the clinical history is a necrobiotic nodule, which can be seen in patients with rheumatoid arthritis (Fig. 5.8). Necrobiotic nodules usually are multiple but occasionally can be solitary. Rheumatoid arthritis is seen more frequently in women than in men, but necrobiotic nodules usually occur in young men and often are associated with subcutaneous nodules. If a necrobiotic nodule is suspected, follow-up films often show the nodule to decrease in size over months to 1 year—and eventually to disappear. Sometimes, a necrobiotic nodule will grow initially, but transthoracic needle biopsy that fails to demonstrate tumor may make it possible to temporize in these patients until the nodule begins decreasing in size.

Solitary Pulmonary Nodule

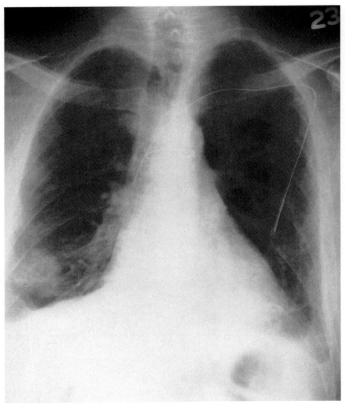

Figure 5.8. Necrobiotic nodule. This 37-year-old man had a necrobiotic nodule in the right lower lobe secondary to rheumatic arthritis. Pleural thickening, also secondary to rheumatoid disease, is present bilaterally.

Developmental Anomalies

Bronchogenic cyst, pulmonary sequestration, and cystic adenomatoid malformation are developmental anomalies that can be quite similar in appearance. They most commonly are seen among children but can occur in any age group, particularly if patients do not have older films to demonstrate this is a congenital lesion.

Bronchogenic Cyst

A bronchogenic cyst is a fairly common mass in the mediastinum, but it is not common in the lung, in which it can be seen as a solitary nodule of almost any size. CT scans show a very homogeneous nodule, and a low HU may be indicative that the nodule is cystic. In many patients with bronchogenic cysts, however, the material in the cyst is highly proteinaceous and causes a high HU, which makes one falsely suspect a tumor.

Pulmonary Sequestration

Pulmonary sequestration (Fig. 5.9) is a developmental anomaly that can present anywhere in the lung, but it usually presents as a mass in the posterior basal segment of one of the lower lobes (more commonly the left). It is characterized by a blood supply from the systemic system, usually directly from the aorta. The supplying vessel generally can be seen on CT scans, MR images, and arteriograms. The sequestration usually is solid but occasionally can be cystic. In general, asymptomatic patients can be followed safely without surgical intervention.

Cystic Adenomatoid Malformation

A developmental anomaly similar to pulmonary sequestration is cystic adenomatoid malformation of the lung, which radiographically often appears similar to pulmonary sequestration. The masses generally are solid but may be cystic. They may contain either fluid or air, and they can vary in size (again like pulmonary sequestration).

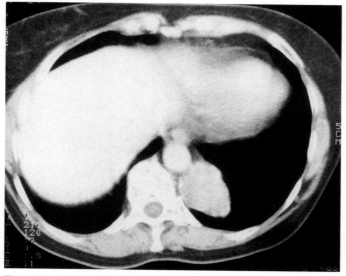

Figure 5.9. Pulmonary sequestration. CT scan shows a rounded mass in the left lower lobe in a 34-year-old woman with history of chronic infections. This finding is consistent with pulmonary sequestration, which was subsequently proved at surgery. A systemic artery supplying the sequestration was not identified on the CT scan but was identified at surgery.

Chapter 5　Solitary Pulmonary Nodule

SUGGESTED READINGS

Bateson EM. An analysis of 155 solitary lung lesions illustrating the differential diagnosis of mixed tumors of the lung. Clin Radiol 1965;16:51–65.

Edwards WM, Cox RS Jr, Garland LH. The solitary nodule (coin lesion) of the lung: an analysis of 52 consecutive cases treated by thoracotomy and a study of preoperative diagnostic accuracy. AJR 1962;88:1020–1042.

Heelan RT, Flehinger BJ, Melamed MR, et al. Non small cell lung cancer: results of the New York screening program. Radiology 1984;151:289–293.

Huston J, Muhm Jr. Solitary pulmonary nodules: evaluation with a CT reference phantom. Radiology 1989;170:653–656.

Muhm JR, Miller WE, Fontana RS, et al. Lung cancer detected during a screening program using 4 month chest radiographs. Radiology 1983;148:609–615.

Nathan MH. Management of solitary pulmonary nodules: an organized approach based on growth rate and statistics. JAMA 1974;227:1141–1144.

O'Keefe ME Jr, Good CA, McDonald JR. Calcification in solitary nodules of the lung. AJR 1957;77:1023–1033.

Siegelman SS, Zerhouni EA, Leo EP, et al. CT of the solitary pulmonary nodule. AJR 1980;135:1–13.

Trunk G, Gracey DR, Byrd RB. The management and evaluation of the solitary pulmonary nodule. Chest 1974;66:236–239.

Multiple Pulmonary Nodules

6

Previous chapters have discussed very tiny nodules (i.e., interstitial lung disease) or ill-defined nodules (i.e., patchy alveolar infiltrates). Like the solitary nodule, multiple pulmonary nodules are well-defined nodular densities in the lungs. There may be two or many, and they may be of varying sizes. They also may be cavitary or noncavitary. Certain diseases are more likely to cause cavitation, but cavitation itself does not significantly change the differential diagnosis.

CAUSES

There are many causes of multiple pulmonary nodules. The most common include:

---

1. Neoplasm.
   A. Metastatic tumor.
   B. Lymphoma.
   C. Posttransplant lymphoproliferative disorder.
   D. Hamartoma.
2. Infection.
   A. Fungal infections.
      i.   Histoplasmosis.
      ii. Coccidioidomycosis.
      iii. Cryptococcosis.
      iv. Invasive aspergillosis.
   B. Bacterial infections.
      i.   Mycobacterial organisms.
      ii. *Nocardia* sp.
      iii. Septic emboli.
3. Parasitic infestation.
4. Arteriovenous malformations.
5. Vasculitis.
6. Bronchiolitis obliterans organizing pneumonia.
7. Necrobiotic nodules.
8. Amyloidosis.

Neoplasms

Metastatic Tumor

By far, metastatic tumor is the most common cause of multiple pulmonary nodules. Almost any tumor can metastasize to the lung, but those that commonly cause pulmonary metastases include breast tumors, kidney tumors, colon tumors, melanomas, testicular tumors, and various sarcomas. Cavitation is not common in patients with metastatic tumors, though it can occur in those undergoing chemotherapy. The most common metastatic tumors in the lung that cavitate are squamous cell tumors, usually from the head and neck or the cervix (Fig. 6.1), but these tumors uncommonly metastasize to the lungs.

Calcification usually does not occur in patients with metastatic tumors, but it may be seen in those with bone- or calcium-forming sarcomas such as osteosarcoma or chondrosarcoma. Calcification in patients with multiple pulmonary nodules usually is suggestive of a nonmalignant diagnosis.

Two or more nodules in the lungs generally are suggestive of metastatic tu-

Chapter 6

Multiple Pulmonary Nodules

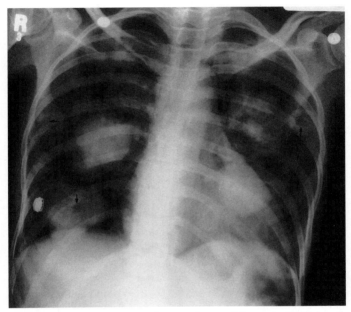

Figure 6.1. Cavitary metastases from carcinoma of the cervix. Multiple pulmonary nodules representing metastatic tumor in a 33-year-old woman with previous carcinoma of the cervix. Several of these nodules are cavitary (*arrows*).

mor. Synchronous primary lung cancers can occur, however, and must be considered when only two or three nodules are identified.

Lymphoma

Lymphoma generally involves the lung as a focal alveolar infiltrate rather than as a true nodule, but occasionally, lymphoma may present as multiple pulmonary nodules. Hodgkin's disease sometimes will appear as multiple well-defined nodules. In addition, lymphomatoid granulomatosis characteristically causes multiple pulmonary nodules. This was once thought to be a benign process that often was a forerunner to lymphoma. Studies with newer histopathologic techniques, however, have shown that lymphomatoid granulomatosis is a true lymphoma. Another lymphomatoid condition that causes multiple pulmonary nodules is pseudolymphoma. This also was once thought to be a benign condition, but in most patients, pseudolymphoma represents a true lymphoma.

Posttransplant Lymphoproliferative Disorder

After organ transplantation, posttransplant lymphoproliferative disorder may occur as solitary or multiple pulmonary nodules (Fig. 6.2). It most commonly is

Multiple Pulmonary Nodules

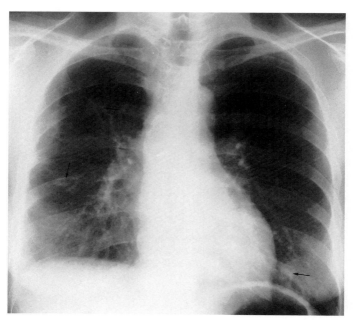

Figure 6.2. Posttransplant lymphoproliferative disorder in a 57-year-old woman. Several ill-defined pulmonary nodules (*arrows*) proved to be posttransplant lymphoproliferative disorder in this patient 1 year after receiving a bilateral lung transplant.

seen in patients who have received lung transplants, but it also can be seen in the lungs of patients who have received other organs. The disorder results from a combination of T-cell immunosuppression and infection with the Epstein-Barr virus. This may have a relatively benign prognosis, disappearing with a decrease in immunosuppressive therapy, or it may develop into an aggressive lymphoma and cause death.

Hamartoma

Benign tumors of the lung are rather uncommon, but one relatively common, benign tumor is hamartoma. A hamartoma is a slow-growing tumor that contains multiple mesenchymal elements. On chest films, it may contain calcification; on computed tomographic (CT) scans, it may contain calcification of mature fat.

Infections

Multiple pulmonary nodules also may result from fungal or bacterial infections.

Chapter 6

Multiple Pulmonary Nodules

Fungal Infections

Histoplasmosis. Fungal infections are the most common infections to present in the lungs as multiple pulmonary nodules, and of these, the most common is histoplasmosis (Fig. 6.3*A,B*). It may be seen as multiple pulmonary nodules that resemble metastatic tumor, and patients frequently are asymptomatic or only mildly symptomatic. The diagnosis can be established on the basis of positive serologic studies for histoplasmosis, but a biopsy often is necessary to be certain that metastatic tumor is not causing the multiple pulmonary nodules. If these nodules are followed over time, they gradually diminish in size and frequently calcify. Multiple calcified nodules scattered throughout the lung fields are highly likely to have resulted from previous histoplasmosis (Fig. 6.3*B*). These infections may occur in the normal host or the immunosupressed patient.

Coccidioidomycosis. A self-limited fungal infection like histoplasmosis, coccidioidomycosis also can produce multiple pulmonary nodules that may proceed to calcification. Coccidioidomycosis causes a chronic infiltrate more com-

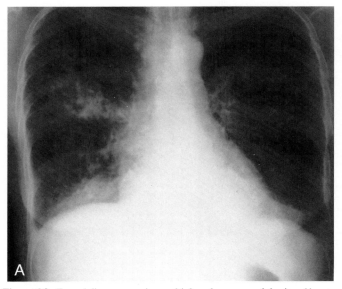

Figure 6.3. Fungal diseases causing multiple pulmonary nodules in a 41-year-old woman. **A.** Histoplasmosis. Multiple small nodules are present throughout both lung fields, and one large right upper lobe nodule is present in this patient with disseminated histoplasmosis. This patient also had chronic liver disease and was receiving steroids. **B.** Histoplasmosis with multiple calcified nodules in a normal host. This is a common finding in geographic areas where histoplasmosis is endemic. **C.** Cryptococcosis. Cryptococcosis with a nodule in the right upper lobe and a less well-defined nodule in the left lower lobe (*arrows*). This patient was a normal host who underwent coronary artery bypass surgery 2 years earlier.

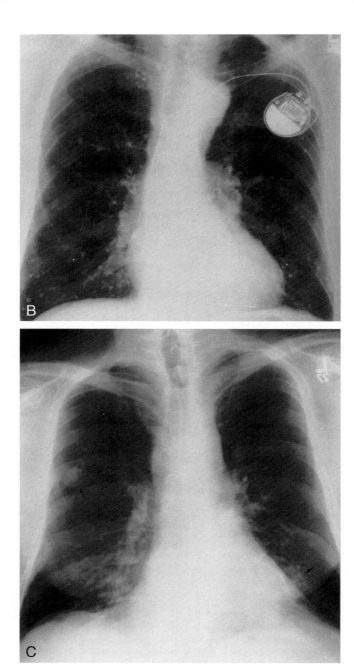

Figure 6.3. (*continued*)

Multiple Pulmonary Nodules

monly than histoplasmosis does, however, and this often takes the form of a solitary cavitary nodule or of multiple nodules, either cavitary or noncavitary. Coccidioidomycosis may cause patchy alveolar infiltrates in the lung as well.

Cryptococcosis. Cryptococcal infection also may cause multiple pulmonary nodules (Fig. 6.3*C*). *Cryptococcus* sp. may affect normal hosts, in which case it is self-limited, but it also has the propensity to affect patients with immunocompromise, particularly those with AIDS. *Cryptococcus* sp. frequently involves the central nervous system, so the combination of multiple pulmonary nodules and central nervous system disease is suggestive of the diagnosis of cryptococcal infection. Of course, metastatic tumor may present in a similar fashion as well.

Invasive Aspergillosis. Invasive aspergillosis occasionally causes pulmonary nodules (Fig. 6.4). Typically, it causes multiple, slightly nodular alveolar infiltrates. The nodular appearance results from invasion of the blood vessels and resultant infarction. These nodules usually are not well circumscribed but on rare occasions may be.

Bacterial Infections

Occasionally, bacterial organisms can cause multiple pulmonary nodules. It is not unusual for bacterial pneumonia to cause a solitary pulmonary nodule (i.e.,

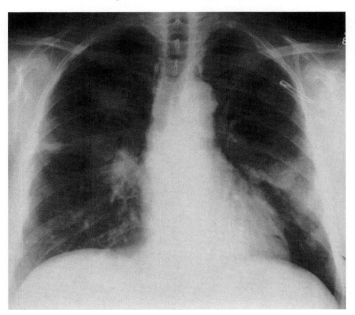

Figure 6.4. Invasive aspergillosis. Multiple, patchy nodular infiltrates are present in both lungs of this 44-year-old male with leukemia. This proved to be invasive aspergillosis.

Multiple Pulmonary Nodules

round pneumonia), but it is unusual for most bacterial agents to cause multiple nodules (except as a septic emboli).

Mycobacterial Organisms. Mycobacterial organisms sometimes may cause multiple pulmonary nodules. In most cases, tuberculosis and the various atypical mycobacterial organisms cause multiple alveolar infiltrates. The various atypical mycobacterial organisms frequently cause bronchiectasis, which may have a somewhat nodular appearance and in turn create the appearance of multiple pulmonary nodules.

Nocardia sp. *Norcardia* sp. will cause solitary or multiple pulmonary nodules in normal hosts and in patients with immunosuppression. More commonly, however, nocardiosis presents as a patchy pneumonia, sometimes with an associated empyema, but it is not unusual for it to occur as single or multiple pulmonary nodules (Fig. 6.5).

Septic Emboli. Septic emboli frequently present as multiple, well-defined pulmonary nodules. They tend to cavitate early (Fig. 6.6), but in some patients,

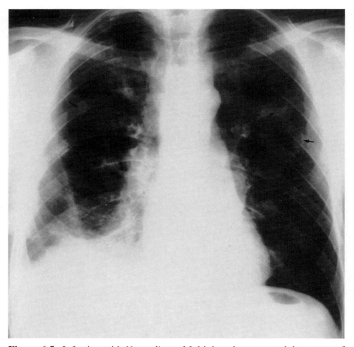

Figure 6.5. Infection with *Nocardia* sp. Multiple pulmonary nodules, many of which are cavitary (*arrows*), are present in this 44-year-old man with AIDS. There also is an associated right pleural effusion. These changes are secondary to nocardiosis.

Multiple Pulmonary Nodules

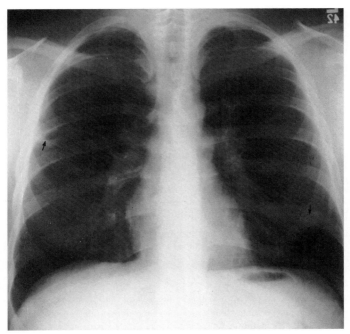

Figure 6.6. Septic emboli. Several cavitary nodules are present (*arrows*) in this 25-year-old male drug abuser. These proved to be septic emboli.

they never cavitate. Septic emboli are always secondary to bacteremia. The source may be indwelling catheters, drug abuse, or various abscesses, including dental abscess. Septic emboli tend to appear rapidly and in patients who are quite ill.

Parasitic Infestations

Parasites are a rare cause of pulmonary nodules in the United States. The most common parasitic cause, however, is hydatid disease *(Echinococcus granulosus)*. Multiple fluid-filled cysts, which appear as pulmonary nodules, can be seen in the lungs. They may have a characteristic peripheral crescent between the true cyst of the parasite and the surrounding pericyst (i.e., a reaction of the body to the parasite). Hydatid disease is a disease of shepherds. The usual hosts are the dog (i.e., intermediate host) and sheep (i.e., primary host), with humans occasionally becoming the primary host as well.

A few other parasitic infestations occasionally cause multiple pulmonary nodules. These include paragonimiasis and schistosomiasis.

Multiple Pulmonary Nodules

Arteriovenous Malformation

Arteriovenous malformations commonly are multiple. They may be confined to the lung or be seen in patients with hereditary telangiectasia (i.e., Rondu-Osler-Weber syndrome) and multiorgan involvement. The diagnosis is readily suggested on the basis of a characteristic, large draining vein on plain films, CT scans, or magnetic resonance images. Embolization of multiple arteriovenous malformations is the usual treatment. Patients are often asymptomatic, but this condition carries a high incidence of brain abscess. Therefore, even asymptomatic patients are treated.

Vasculitis

Most vasculitides do not cause well-circumscribed nodules in the lung. Occasionally, however, they can, especially in patients with Wegener's granulomatosis. Churg-Strauss vasculitis and bronchocentric granulomatosis also may cause well-circumscribed nodules.

Bronchiolitis Obliterand Organizing Pneumonia

Bronchiolitis obliterans organizing pneumonia typically causes patchy alveolar infiltrates. Occasionally, however, it may cause solitary or multiple well-circumscribed nodules.

Necrobiotic Nodules

Another rare cause of multiple nodules is rheumatoid arthritis. Necrobiotic nodules usually are encountered in young men early in the course of disease. Of course, rheumatoid arthritis is more common among women, but these patients have necrobiotic nodules less frequently.

Amyloidosis

Another rare cause of multiple pulmonary nodules (sometimes calcified) is amyloidosis. Calcification in pulmonary nodules also may be a sequela of primary infection. This is especially true of histoplasmosis but occasionally may be seen with coccidioidomycosis, varicella, or measles as well.

SUGGESTED READINGS

Albelda SM, Kern JA, Marinelli DL, et al. Expanding spectrum of pulmonary disease caused by nontuberculous mycobacteria. Radiology 1985;157:289–296.

Coppage L, Shaw C, McBride-Curtis A. Metastatic disease to the chest in patients with extrathoracic malignancy. J Thorac Imaging 1987;2:24–37.

Crow J, Slavin G, Kreel L. Pulmonary metastases: a pathologic and radiologic study. Cancer 1981;47:2595–2602.

Godwin JD, Webb WR, Savoca CJ, Gamsu GP. Multiple thin walled cystic lesions of the lung. AJR 1980;135:593–604.

Goodwin RA, Loyd JE, Des Prez RM. Histoplasmosis in normal hosts. Medicine 1981;60:231.

Miller WT, ed. Fungus diseases of the chest. Semin Roentgenol. Philadelphia: WB Saunders. Vol XXXl, 1996.

Miller WT. Granulomatous infections of the lung. In: Freundlich IM, Bragg DG, eds. A radiologic approach to diseases of the chest. Baltimore: Williams & Wilkins, 1992:263–287.

Rippon SW. Medical mycology: the pathogenic fungi and the pathogenic actinomycetes. 3rd ed. Philadelphia: WB Saunders, l988.

Zimmerman RA, Miller WT. Pulmonary aspergillosis. AJR l970;l09:505–515.

Hyperlucency of the Lungs 7

Hyperlucency of the lungs can be diffuse or focal. Usually, it is diffuse and secondary to emphysema (Fig. 7.1).

CAUSES

Causes of hyperlucency of the lungs include:

1. Diffuse.
   A. Chronic obstructive pulmonary disease
      i. Emphysema.
      ii. Asthma.
2. Focal.
   A. Congenital problems associated with focal emphysema.
   B. Bullae.
   C. Idiopathic bullous disease.
   D. Blebs.

Diffuse Hyperlucency of the Lungs

Chronic Obstructive Pulmonary Disease

The difficulty in distinguishing between the various causes of obstructive airway disease has led to the clinical term *chronic obstructive pulmonary disease* (COPD) or *chronic obstructive lung disease* (COLD). This is an all-encompassing diagnosis that includes emphysema, chronic bronchitis, asthma, bronchiectasis, and bronchiolitis obliterans. Frequently, one patient may actually have several of these diseases. Chronic obstructive pulmonary disease is a general and not a specific term; therefore, it should not be used to imply the presence of any specific disease.

Emphysema. Emphysema is a pathologic abnormality of the lung that destroys alveoli and results in obstruction of small airways. Alveolar destruction can be divided on the basis of morphology into three types: centrilobular, panlobular, and paraseptal emphysema.

In centrilobular emphysema, there is incomplete destruction of the lung distal to the terminal bronchiole. The destruction tends to occur in the center of the lobule but may be eccentric. This type of emphysema is the most common and usually is secondary to smoking.

In panlobular emphysema, there is complete destruction of the lung distal to the terminal bronchiole. This type of emphysema is frequently congenital and secondary to α_1-antitrypsin deficiency. Panlobular emphysema tends to involve the lower lobes more than the upper lobes (Fig. 7.2).

Figure 7.1. Emphysema. Posteroanterior (**A**) and lateral (**B**) chest films show severe hyperinflation of the lung fields caused by emphysema. The vessels are stretched and bullous changes are present, particularly in the right upper lobe. The lateral film (**B**) shows flattening of the diaphragm. The posteroanterior film (**A**) shows chronic changes in the left upper lobe that represent scarring from a prevous pneumonia.

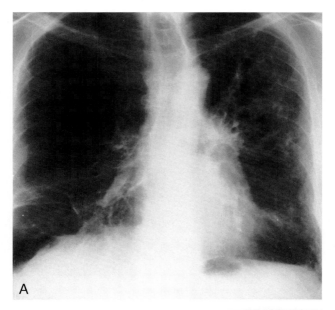

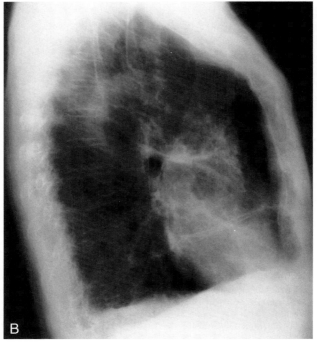

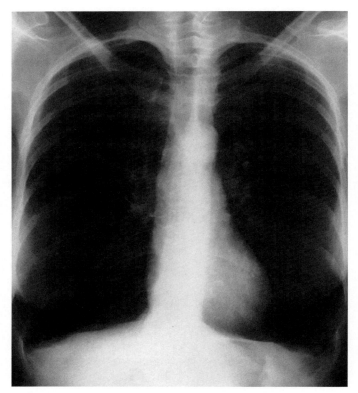

Figure 7.2. α_1-Antitrypsin deficiency with panlobular emphysema. This 33-year-old woman had diffuse pulmonary emphysema, which was most marked at the lung bases. This is characteristic of α_1-antitrypsin deficiency.

Paraseptal emphysema appears radiographically as a peripheral, subpleural distribution of emphysema. This may be seen in association with centrilobular emphysema, or it can be an isolated idiopathic disorder. The idiopathic form is seen in younger adult patients and is associated with giant bullae as well as with an increased incidence of spontaneous pneumothorax.

The plain chest film is not very sensitive in the detection of emphysema. The usual findings are hyperinflation of the lung fields, flattening of the diaphragm, increased retrosternal space, and decreased heart size. Of these indicators for emphysema, flattening of the diaphragm is the most reliable. All of the these criteria are not very sensitive to the presence of emphysema in the lungs, however, and they also are not very specific. For example, hyperinflation of the lung frequently occurs in thin individuals who make a good inspiratory effort that may mimic emphysema.

Hyperlucency of the Lungs

When present, vascular destruction is a fairly specific indicator for emphysema. Vascular destruction causes the vessels to be stretched or absent in portions of the lung fields. If bullae are present, the vessels may be crowded together in more normal areas where bullae are not present.

Computed tomography (particularly high-resolution computed tomography) is extremely useful in detecting the early morphologic changes of emphysema. It is also useful in recognizing the various types of emphysema (Fig. 7.3).

Asthma. Another cause of diffuse hyperlucency of the lungs is status asthmaticus. Asthma does not cause chronic hyperinflation of the lung, but in patients undergoing severe asthmatic attacks, bronchospasm traps air, which in turn causes hyperinflation of the lung fields and decreases the size of the pulmonary vessels. When the asthma is controlled, however, the hyperinflation disappears.

In older patients with "asthma," there may be hyperinflation of the lung fields. Such patients probably have emphysema with a bronchospastic or asthmatic component and are not solely asthmatics.

Focal Hyperlucency of the Lungs

Congenital Problems

Congenital lobar emphysema is an anomaly that may lead to severe hyperlucency of part or all of one lung. This disease occurs in newborns and tends to disappear as patients age (Fig. 7.4). Other congenital lesions that occasionally

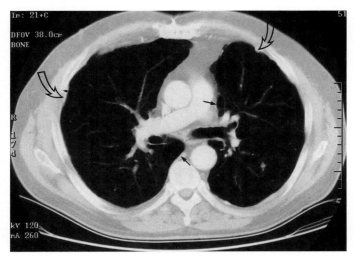

Figure 7.3. Centrilobular and paraseptal emphysema and pleural plaques. Scattered lucencies are seen throughout both lungs that represent centrilobular emphysema. Peripheral bullae also are seen along both sides of the mediastinum (*closed arrows*) that represent paraseptal emphysema. In addition, note the characteristic pleural plaques (*open arrows*) from previous exposure to asbestos.

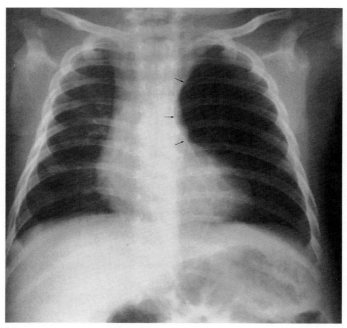

Figure 7.4. Congenital lobar emphysema of the left upper lobe. Note the hyperlucency of the left upper lobe (*arrows*) with a shift of the mediastinum to the right.

cause a lucent defect within the lung are those that usually are filled with fluid but occasionally can be filled with air: bronchogenic cyst, pulmonary sequestration, and cystic adenomatoid malformation of the lung.

Bullae

A bulla is a collection of air within the lung and represents a distended secondary pulmonary lobule or group of lobules. Bullae may be as small as several centimeters or large enough to fill an entire hemithorax almost completely (Fig. 7.5).

Bullae are frequent accompaniments of centrilobular emphysema. They can occur anywhere in the lung but are more frequent in the upper lobes. Over time, bullae tend to enlarge and push the normal lung aside. Currently popular, lung reduction surgery is best suited for patients with several or many large bullae, a very heterogeneous distribution of emphysema, or both throughout the lungs.

Hyperlucency of the Lungs

Idiopathic Bullous Disease

A disease of smokers, centrilobular emphysema is generally seen in patients 50 years of age and older. Occasionally, a type of bullous emphysema occurs in younger patients, who are sometimes in their early thirties and frequently in their late thirties and early forties (Fig. 7.6). This is usually associated with paraseptal emphysema, where one or a few of the peripheral air spaces enlarge into giant bullae that compress the adjacent lung (Fig. 7.5). The remaining portion of the lung not involved in the bullae may be relatively normal. These patients usually are heavy smokers, but they also probably have a congenital predisposition to the development of bullae. They are ideally suited for bullectomy or lung reduction surgery.

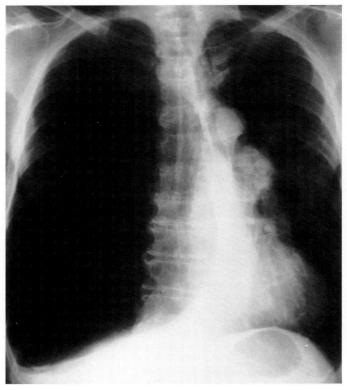

Figure 7.5. Large bulla in the right lung. This 47-year-old man had a large bulla on the right that displaced the mediastinum to the left. No vascular markings are seen on the right. This bulla should not be mistaken for a pneumothorax, because there is no evidence of collapsed lung in the area of the right hilum.

Hyperlucency of the Lungs Chapter 7

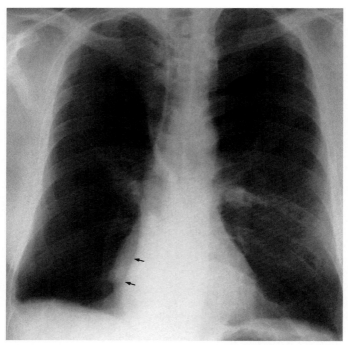

Figure 7.6. Idiopathic bullous lung disease. This 37-year-old man had extensive bullae throughout the right lung and the left upper lobe that obliterated the vascular markings in this area. Note that the right lower lobe is collapsed against the mediastinum (*arrows*).

Blebs. A bleb is a collection of air just beneath the visceral pleura of the lung. Closely related to the bleb is the subpleural air cyst or pneumatocele. In patients undergoing assisted ventilation, the increased airway pressures may rupture a small bronchus. When this happens, the air can dissect centrally along the bronchovascular bundles and cause mediastinal emphysema (a common occurrence). Alternatively, the air can dissect peripherally and create a subpleural air cyst or pneumatocele. This is significantly less common than development of mediastinal emphysema, and these subpleural air cysts may rupture and create a pneumothorax.

In patients with pneumonia, and particularly in children with staphylococcal pneumonia, a small bronchus occasionally may rupture in the area of the pneumonia, with dissection of the air subpleurally and creation of a subpleural air cyst or pneumatocele. This pneumatocele frequently is filled with fluid or with air and fluid, but it should not be confused with a lung abscess. The pneumatocele has a much more benign prognosis than a lung abscess.

Blunt trauma may create a shearing force in the lung that results in laceration of the lung parenchyma. This laceration then fills with air, fluid, or both, and it has the appearance of a cyst or pneumatocele (Fig. 7.7). As with other causes of

Hyperlucency of the Lungs

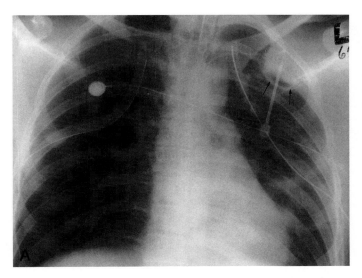

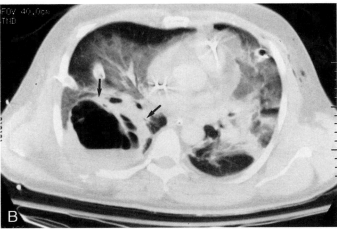

Figure 7.7. Pulmonary laceration. **A.** Posteroanterior film of a 20-year-old man with a left upper lobe laceration (*arrows*) partially filled by fluid. There also is a contusion of the left lower lobe. **B.** Computed tomographic scan of a 18-year-old man with a right lower lobe laceration (*arrows*) that resembles a lung abscess. A prominent air-fluid level is present. This patient also had adult respiratory distress syndrome, with patchy consolidation in both lungs.

pneumatocele, this should not be confused with a lung abscess, because the prognosis for a pulmonary laceration is much better.

SUGGESTED READINGS

Bergin C, Muller N, Nichols DM, et al. The diagnosis of emphysema: a computed tomographic-pathologic correlation. Am Rev Respir Dis 1986;133:541–546.

Dines DE. Diagnostic significance of pneumatocele of the lung. JAMA 1968;204:1169–1172.

Gerblich AA, Kleinerman J. Blunt chest trauma and the lung. Am Rev Respir Dis 1977;115:369–370.

Heitzman RB: Chronic obstructive pulmonary disease. In: Heitzman RB, ed. The lung: radiologic-pathologic correlation. 2nd ed. St. Louis: CV Mosby, 1984;429–456.

Kerns Sr, Gay SB. CT of blunt chest trauma. AJR 1990;154:55–60.

Kinsella M, Muller NL, Staples C, Vedl S, Chan-Yeung M. Hyperinflation in asthma and emphysema: assessment by pulmonary function testing and computed tomography. Chest 1988;94:286–289.

Pratt PC. Role of conventional chest radiography in diagnosis and exclusion of emphysema. Am J Med 1987;82:998–1006.

Reid L. The pathology of emphysema. London: Lloyd-Luke, 1967.

Sefczek DM, Defczek RJ, Dash N, Shapiro RL. Lucent lesions of the lung. Postgrad Radiol 1987;7:139–156.

Snider GL, Kleinerman J, Thurlbeck WM, Bengali ZH. The definition of emphysema. Report of a National Heart, Lung and Blood Institute, Division of Lung Diseases Workshop. Am Rev Respir Dis 1985;132:182–185.

Thurlbeck WM, Henderson JA, Fraser RG, Bates DV. Chronic obstructive lung disease: a comparison between clinical, roentgenologic, functional and morphologic criteria in chronic bronchitis, emphysema, asthma and bronchiectasis. Medicine 1970;49:82–145.

8

Pleura

The pleura can be affected by various disease processes. In most cases, a pleural effusion or collection of fluid results between the parietal and the visceral pleura. In others, diffuse pleural thickening, fibrosis, or pleural nodulation may result.

PLEURAL EFFUSION

The role of the radiologist in pleural effusion is, first and foremost, to recognize pleural fluid. In this matter, the radiologist is primary. He or she plays only a minor role, however, in determining the cause of a pleural effusion, though the radiologist can often make an educated guess.

Recognition of Pleural Fluid

Free pleural fluid collects in the dependent portions of the pleural space. In upright or ambulatory patients, these portions are at the bases of the lung. Because of both the small size of the pleural space and the capillary action of fluids, pleural effusion tends to cause a meniscus at the borders of the lung (Fig. 8.1). This meniscus characteristically is seen in the lateral costophrenic angle, but it also may be seen in the medial and posterior costophrenic angles (Figs. 8.2 and 8.3).

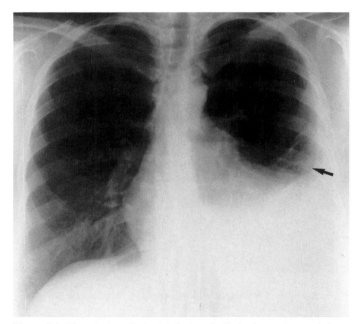

Figure 8.1. Pleural tuberculosis. A left pleural effusion has a characteristic meniscus (*arrow*). This effusion was secondary to primary tuberculosis in a 30-year-old man.

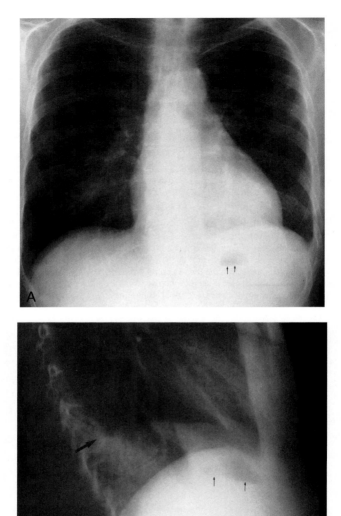

Figure 8.2. Left pleural effusion caused by viral pleuritis. This 22-year-old man had minimal blunting of the left costophrenic sulcus on the posteroanterior film (**A**). The lateral film (**B**) shows obvious blunting of the left costophrenic sulcus posteriorly by the pleural effusion (*closed arrow*). The right costophrenic angle is not blunted (*open arrow*). The stomach bubble (*small arrows*) is separated from the lung on both films, indicating a subpulmonic collection of fluid.

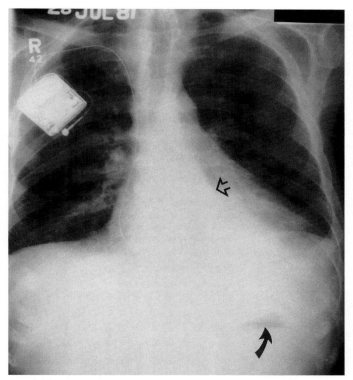

Figure 8.3. Subpulmonic effusion secondary to congestive failure. The left costophrenic angle is not blunted, but a density behind the heart resembles left lower lobe atelectasis but is actually a medial meniscus from the left pleural effusion (*open arrow*). The stomach bubble (*closed arrow*) is considerably displaced from the lung, indicating a large subpulmonic effusion on the left and a smaller pleural effusion on the right.

The posterior costophrenic sulcus is the most inferior sulcus, so it is the first sulcus to fill with fluid on the upright chest film. Thus, the lateral film is key in recognition of a small pleural effusion. From 30 to 50 mL of fluid may blunt the posterior costophrenic sulcus (Fig. 8.2), but several hundred milliliters frequently are required to blunt the lateral costophrenic sulcus. In some patients, there may be no blunting of the lateral costophrenic sulcus, only of the medial costophrenic sulcus, so the radiologist must be able to recognize fluid in this area as well (Fig. 8.3).

For unknown reasons, some patients with pleural effusions tend to collect fluid beneath the lung (i.e., subpulmonic effusion) and also maintain the shape of the lung (Fig. 8.3). There are several clues to the presence of subpulmonic effusion. For example, the posterior costophrenic sulcus usually, but not always, is blunted (Fig. 8.2). One also usually recognizes the location of the diaphragm by aerated lung above the diaphragm. In a subpulmonic effusion, however, the lung is not adjacent to the diaphragm. The true location of the diaphragm may be recognized by air in the stomach on the left side (Figs. 8.2 and 8.3) and occasionally by free air under the diaphragm, which may fortuitously help to identify a subpulmonic effusion.

In the supine position commonly used in the intensive care unit, large amounts of fluid may accumulate in the pleural space and go unrecognized. This fluid accumulates posterior to the lung; therefore, it does not blunt the costophrenic angle. If different amounts of fluid are in the two pleural spaces, the side with the most fluid may appear to be more opaque on the chest film. Care must be taken when using this sign, however, because rotating the patient also will produce different densities in the two hemithoraces. The most specific evidence of fluid behind the lung is the meniscus of fluid at the apex and the lateral aspects of the lung (Fig. 8.4), but this occurs only in very large pleural effusions. Computed tomography (CT) is of great help in recognizing pleural effusions in critically ill patients in the intensive care unit.

The decubitus film is paramount in establishing that a blunted costophrenic sulcus is caused by free pleural fluid and not by pleural thickening or a loculated

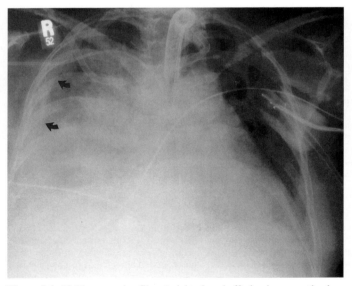

Figure 8.4. Fluid on a supine film. A right pleural effusion increases the density of the right hemithorax. A meniscus can be seen along the lateral chest wall (*arrows*).

pleural effusion On a decubitus film, free fluid appears as an opaque band between the lung and the lateral surface of the ribs.

Loculation of pleural effusion occurs when the fluid contains a large amount of protein. This is most common in malignant, infectious (Figs. 8.5 and 8.6), or traumatic effusions (i.e., hemothorax). Fluid can loculate in any portion of the pleural space, but it tends to loculate in a dependent location. Thus, the fluid frequently is loculated posteriorly, because ill patients often are supine. If patients are ambulatory, the fluid tends to loculate at the lung bases. As mentioned, a decubitus film will differentiate between free and loculated fluid.

Fluid also may collect in the major and minor fissures between the lungs, and fluid in these fissures may be either free or loculated. Such fluid may create a round shadow that resembles a pulmonary mass (i.e., pseudotumor) (Fig. 8.7A). On a lateral film, the shape of the "mass" usually is lenticular or cigar-shaped, which confirms that the mass is a pleural pseudotumor (Fig. 8.7B).

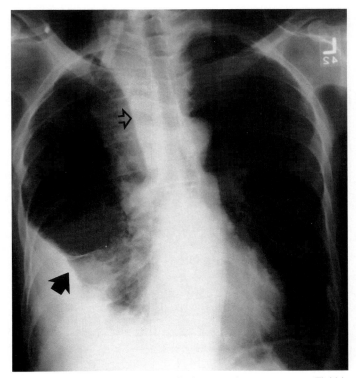

Figure 8.5. Loculated right pleural effusion secondary to empyema. Fluid is loculated medially about the upper mediastinum (*open arrow*) and at the right base (*closed arrow*) secondary to empyema.

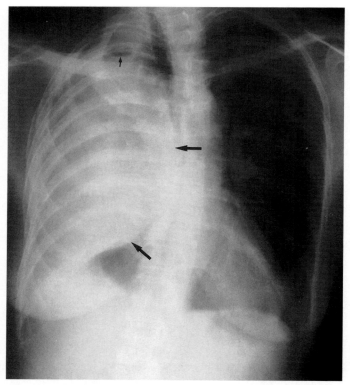

Figure 8.6. Loculated pleural effusion secondary to tuberculosis. This 60-year-old woman had a large, loculated right pleural effusion (*large arrows*). This represents primary tuberculosis. A small air-fluid level at the right apex (*small arrow*) indicates a bronchopleural fistula.

Causes

There are many causes of pleural effusion. The most common include:

1. Congestive heart failure.
2. Infection.
   A. Parapneumonic.
   B. Tuberculous.
   C. Viral pleuritis.
   D. Fungal.

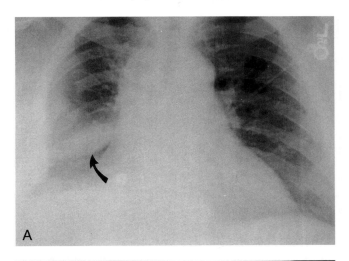

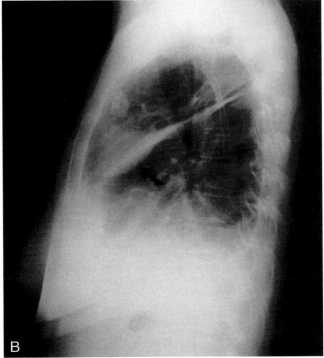

Figure 8.7. Loculated pleural effusion creating a phantom tumor. Fluid in the right major fissure is round and suggests a lung mass (*arrow*) on the posteroanterior film (**A**). On the lateral film (**B**), the collection is lens-shaped (*arrow*).

> 3. Tumor.
>   A. Metastases.
>   B. Lymphoma.
>   C. Mesothelioma.
> 4. Collagen vascular disease.
> 5. Trauma.
>   A. Esophageal rupture.
> 6. Subdiaphragmatic process.
>   A. Abdominal surgery.
>   B. Subphrenic abscess.
> 7. Previous surgery.

Congestive Heart Failure

By far, congestive heart failure is the most common cause of pleural effusion. If the patient has bilateral pleural effusions and those effusions are not loculated, congestive heart failure usually is the cause—even if the heart is not enlarged. Generally, however, the heart is enlarged in patients with effusions secondary to congestive failure.

Infection

Parapneumonic. Pneumonia often is accompanied by a pleural effusion (i.e., parapneumonic). This effusion usually does not contain organisms, but if it does, an empyema may develop. Most parapneumonic effusions are not loculated. An empyema usually is, though, because it is high in protein.

In most patients with a parapneumonic effusion, pneumonia will be evident. Some patients may have an established empyema, however, and no apparent pneumonia.

Tuberculous. A tuberculous infection usually occurs in patients with no evidence of a pulmonary infiltrate. Tuberculous effusions generally are unilateral.

Viral Pleuritis. Viral pleuritis also usually occurs in patients with no evidence of a pulmonary infiltrate. Viral pleuritis frequently is bilateral and often is accompanied by pericarditis, but it also may be unilateral. Viral pleuritis is not very common, but it should be suspected in febrile patients with an unexplained exudative effusion.

Fungal. Fungal infections do not commonly cause pleural effusions. Fungal empyema occasionally may be seen, however, with almost any fungal infection. Several chronic bacterial infections (i.e., actinomycosis or nocardiosis) also may cause a pleural effusion.

Tumor

Metastases. Metastatic tumors are a very common cause of an exudative pleural effusion. Such tumors may be bilateral but more commonly are unilateral. Breast and lung cancer are the two most common causes of metastatic effusions, but almost any tumor sometimes may cause a metastatic pleural effusion.

Lymphoma. Lymphoma sometimes can present with a pleural effusion as the only finding. This is fairly common among patients with AIDS but also can occur in other patients as well. Generally, pleural effusion occurs with known lymphoma.

Mesothelioma. Mesothelioma is a highly malignant tumor of the pleura that usually presents as a pleural effusion. During the later stages, it usually is loculated and has a very lumpy or nodular appearance. The tumor is always diffuse, though it rarely may start with local involvement of the chest wall. It usually involves only one pleural space. As a later manifestation, however, it involves the chest wall and may metastasize to the mediastinum, lungs, or abdominal organs (Fig. 8.8).

Collagen Vascular Disease

Lupus erythematosus and rheumatoid arthritis are the two collagen vascular diseases that commonly cause pleural effusions. These effusions usually are exudative and bilateral, and they often are loculated. Many drugs can create a lupus reaction that may be almost indistinguishable from idiopathic lupus. Most common among these are procainamide, Isoniazid, hydralizine, and Dilantin.

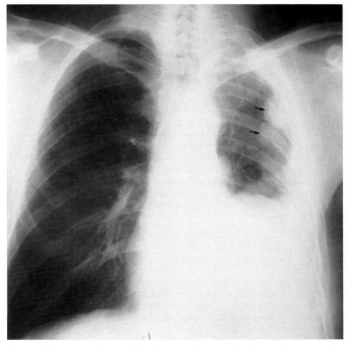

Figure 8.8. Mesothelioma. This 67-year-old man had a large left pleural effusion. Multiple pleural nodules (*arrows*) indicate the malignant nature of this effusion. This could be either metastatic tumor or mesothelioma, but it proved to be the latter.

Pleura

Trauma

Pleural effusion commonly accompanies various types of trauma. It occurs with blunt trauma to the chest from motor vehicle accidents and in penetrating trauma from a gunshot or stab wound. It also occurs in postoperative patients after surgical trauma to the lungs or mediastinum. If fluid is seen to accumulate rapidly, a hemothorax must be suspected.

Esophageal Rupture. Esophageal rupture is an important traumatic event that is quite difficult to diagnose and frequently is overlooked. A small left pleural effusion may be a clue to the presence of this life-threatening event. Esophageal rupture generally occurs in patients, particularly those with alcoholism, who have been vomiting or retching.

Subdiaphragmatic Process

Abdominal Surgery. Various intraabdominal conditions may cause pleural effusion, and abdominal ascites is one such common cause. In ascites, fluid passes from the peritoneum through tiny holes in the diaphragm into the chest. The effusion can be unilateral on either side, or it can be bilateral in patients with small or large amounts of ascites.

Subphrenic Abscess. Subphrenic abscess usually is accompanied by pleural effusion on the side of that abscess. Inflammatory processes in the abdomen, such as pancreatitis and occasionally cholecystitis, also may have an associated pleural effusion.

Previous Surgery

An important cause of pleural effusion that a radiologist should recognize as being benign is previous surgery. Pleural effusion may be associated with abdominal, thoracic, or neck surgery. This effusion usually is small, however, and disappears rapidly as the patient recovers from the surgery. Even so, after heart surgery with a pericardiotomy, a pleural effusion may persist for many months. Benign effusions after a pericardiotomy have been reported as long as 1 year after the surgery. Similarly, a pleural effusion may occur several weeks to months after a myocardial infarction or pericardiotomy and is known as Dressler's syndrome (after an infarct) or postpericardiotomy syndrome (after surgery). This type of effusion usually is self-limited.

PLEURAL NODULES OR MASSES

Recognition

A pleural nodule may be difficult to distinguish from an extrapleural (i.e., chest wall) nodule or mass. The shape of both pleural and chest wall masses often is identical: a very smooth mass with tapering edges when seen in profile (Fig. 8.9). The mass tends to have its greatest diameter at the midportion of the mass (see Fig. 9.5) and also to have tapering (i.e., acute) margins. Extrapleural masses or chest wall lesions almost always invade the bony structures, particularly the ribs. If a pleural or extrapleural mass is suspected, adjacent bony structures should be examined carefully, because bony involvement is suggestive of an extrapleural location.

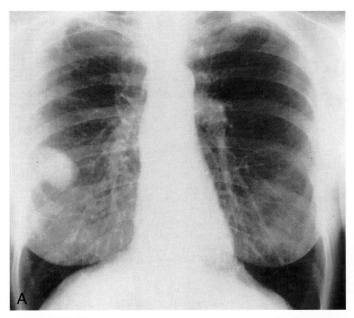

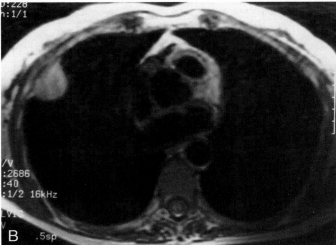

Figure 8.9. Metastatic pleural nodule caused by ovarian carcinoma. The pleural nature of the mass in this 60-year-old woman is only indicated on the posteroanterior film (**A**), because the medial portion of the nodule is sharp but the lateral portion is indistinct. A magnetic resonance image (**B**) shows the pleural nature of this mass.

111

Pleura

Causes

Most pleural nodules or masses are secondary to neoplasms (Fig. 8.9). In most patients, this is a metastatic tumor, and even a solitary mass should make one suspect a metastatic tumor. The most common benign causes of a solitary mass are pleural fibroma and pleural lipoma. Multiple pleural masses are strongly suggestive of primary or metastatic tumor of the pleura. Multiple masses must be distinguished from loculated pleural fluid, however, which may be identical in appearance. Loculated fluid sometimes can simulate a solitary pleural mass as well, but there usually are other indications that pleural fluid is present. Therefore, a loculated effusion can be suspected. Infection or other inflammatory masses can cause loculated pleural effusion and sometimes create the appearance of multiple pleural masses. Generally, inflammatory problems cause large loculations rather than the small loculations, the later of which might simulate pleural nodules.

Many tumors can metastasize to the pleura and cause pleural nodules, but breast carcinoma probably is the most common metastatic tumor. Primary pleural mesothelioma, particularly during its later stages, also frequently causes pleural nodulation. Most tumors that cause pleural nodulation also cause an associated pleural effusion at the same time (Fig. 8.8). One tumor that usually does not cause a pleural effusion, however, is metastatic thymoma. In some patients, metastatic pleural nodules may be the only clue to the presence of a malignant thymoma. The primary tumor may be occult in the mediastinum or on the chest film, but it often is easily demonstrated by CT, which also can help to differentiate between loculated pleural fluid and a solid pleural tumor.

If multiple nodules are all in one hemithorax, this is strongly suggestive of a pleural rather than a pulmonary cause for the nodules. It also usually indicates metastatic tumor to the pleura.

The major benign cause of multiple pleural nodules is asbestos-related pleural plaques (Fig. 8.10). These are the most common manifestation of asbestos exposure and usually occur seen from 15 to 20 years after the exposure. Unlike pleural tumors, they are almost always bilateral. They may calcify 30 to 40 years after the primary exposure, but the early pleural plaques are noncalcified. Calcification usually clinches the diagnosis of pleural plaques. Unlike neoplastic pleural thickening, which usually has a rounded contour, pleural plaques may have a characteristic plateau shape when seen in profile, particularly on CT scans. This usually is not obvious, however, on the plain chest film.

Occasionally, it may be difficult to differentiate peripheral lung nodules from a pleural nodule or mass. This is particularly true for carcinoma of the lung, which also can resemble pleural thickening at the lung apex. Asymmetrical pleural thickening is always suggestive of possible lung carcinoma (i.e., Pancoast tumor) (Fig. 8.11).

PLEURAL CALCIFICATION

Unilateral pleural calcification usually is associated with pleural thickening in the involved hemithorax, which also causes blunting of the costophrenic angle. Unilateral pleural thickening and calcification generally are secondary to previous tuberculosis, empyema, or hemothorax (Fig. 8.12). Calcification frequently is extensive, and the pleural thickening may be mild to extensive.

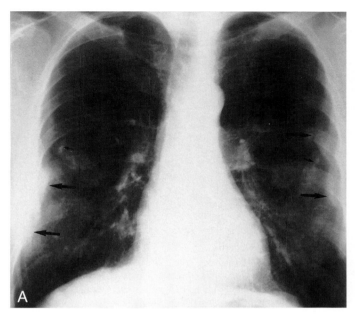

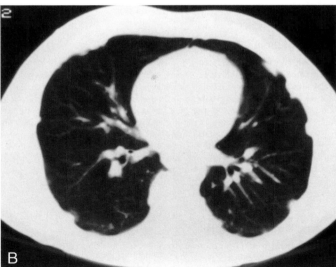

Figure 8.10. Multiple pleural nodules secondary to asbestos exposure. **A.** This 62-year-old man has multiple bilateral pleural nodules (*arrows*). Calcification can be seen in several of the nodules (*small arrows*). **B.** CT scan shows the characteristic pleural location of these nodules and a shelf-like pattern (see also Fig. 7.3).

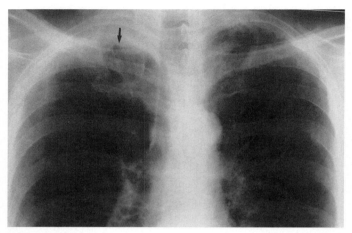

Figure 8.11. Pancoast tumor. This 70-year-old man appeared to have asymmetrical pleural thickening, with the right side being more thickened than the left (*arrow*). This appearance should make one suspect a primary carcinoma of the lung (Pancoast tumor), which this case proved to be.

Unilateral Pleural Calcification

Unilateral pleural thickening may occur without pleural calcification and usually relates to one of the three causes mentioned earlier (i.e., tuberculosis, empyema, or hemothorax). Other exudative effusions such as collagen vascular disease, previous benign asbestos effusion, previous pulmonary infarction, and primary or metastatic tumor may cause unilateral pleural thickening as well. Tumor generally causes a pleural effusion and pleural nodulation. This is particularly true for metastatic tumor and usually true for mesothelioma as well. Rarely, however, pleural mesothelioma may cause focal pleural thickening in its early stages, and it may have a very benign appearance. A clue to mesothelioma in this case is that previous, recent films do not show the pleural thickening and that the patient often complains of chest wall pain. In this situation, focal pleural thickening is an ominous sign.

Bilateral Pleural Calcification

Bilateral pleural calcification rarely is caused by tuberculosis, previous empyema, or hemothorax. These are unilateral conditions. Bilateral pleural calcification usually is caused by asbestos exposure. The pleural calcifications may be minimal or extensive, and they characteristically involve the domes of the diaphragm. Pleural calcification occurs 30 to 40 years after the asbestos exposure and may be seen in CT scans only when noncalcified pleural plaques are identified on the plain chest films. CT scans also may show pleural plaques that were not visible on the plain films.

Pleura

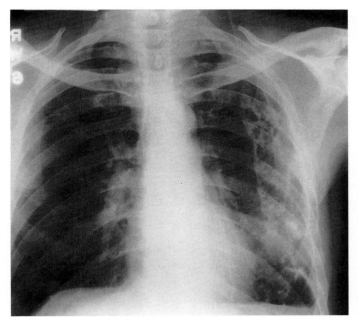

Figure 8.12. Left fibrothorax. The left costophrenic sulcus is blunted by pleural thickening, and there is fairly extensive pleural calcification overlying the left chest wall. This fibrothorax was secondary to primary tuberculosis.

SELECTED READINGS

England DM, Hochholzer L, McCarthy MJ. Localized benign and malignant fibrous tumors of the pleura. Am J Surg Pathol 1989;13:640–658.

Fleischner FG. Atypical arrangement of free pleural effusion. Radiol Clin North Am 1963;1:347–362.

Henschke C, Davis S, Yankelevitz D, Romano P. The pathogenesis, radiologic evaluation, and therapy of pleural effusions. Radiol Clin North Am 1989;27:1241–1255.

Moller A. Pleural effusion: use of the semi-supine position for radiographic detection. Radiology 1984;150:245–249.

Petersen JA. Recognition of infrapulmonary pleural effusion. Radiology 1960;74:34–41.

Pugatch RD, Faling LJ, Robbins AH, Snider GL. Differentation of pleural and pulmonary lesions using computed tomography. J Comput Assist Tomogr 1978;2:601–606.

Sahebjami H, Loudon RG. Pleural effusions: pathophysiology and clinical features. Semin Roentgenol 1977;12:269–275.

Stark DD, Federle MP, Goodman PC, et al. Differentiating lung abscess and empyema: radiography and computed tomography. AJR 1983;141:163–167.

Diaphragm and Chest Wall   9

THE DIAPHRAGM

The diaphragm is the paramount muscle in respiration. The most important abnormalities involving the diaphragm relate to its movement. The finding at chest x-ray that indicates poor movement of the diaphragm is usually elevation of the diaphragm, either bilateral or unilateral.

Bilateral Elevation

The most common cause of bilateral diaphragmatic elevation is obesity. When patients inspire, the diaphragm must move downward, but if the abdomen is distended by some process, this distension impedes the downward motion of the diaphragm. The most common cause of abdominal distention is fat. The abdomen also can be distended by ascites, however, or by organomegaly such as an enlarged liver, spleen, kidney, or uterus.

Another cause of bilateral diaphragmatic elevation is abdominal or chest pain with resultant splinting of the diaphragm. This frequently occurs during the postoperative period. In addition, bilateral diaphragmatic paralysis is a rare cause of bilateral diaphragmatic elevation.

Unilateral Elevation

Causes of unilateral diaphragmatic elevation include:

1. Diminished pulmonary volume.
   A. Atelectasis.
   B. Lobectomy.
2. Phrenic nerve paralysis.
3. Eventration of the diaphragm.
4. Intraabdominal process.
   A. Organomegaly.
   B. Subphrenic abscess.
5. Subpulmonic effusion.

Diminished Pulmonary Volume

Unilateral diaphragmatic elevation is a secondary sign of atelectasis and may be seen in patients with very tight lobar atelectasis. Previous lobectomy also will diminish lung volume and may cause an elevated hemidiaphragm. This is particularly true if the patient has undergone bilobectomy.

Phrenic Nerve Paralysis

Surgery also may cause diaphragmatic elevation by involving the phrenic nerve and is the most common cause of diaphragmatic paralysis. The phrenic nerve may be injured either directly during neck or chest surgery or indirectly by cardioplegic fluids used in heart surgery or cooling fluid used in lung transplantation, with resultant temporary phrenic nerve paralysis. In patients with no previous surgery, diaphragmatic paralysis usually is secondary to phrenic nerve involvement by a mediastinal mass (usually a malignant tumor).

Fluoroscopy of the chest is the best way to evaluate patients for diaphragmatic paralysis. This is because the paralyzed diaphragm moves paradoxically on breathing.

Eventration of the Diaphragm

The most common cause of diaphragmatic elevation is eventration of the diaphragm (Fig. 9.1). This process involves loss of or weakness in a portion of the diaphragmatic muscle, and in some patients, it may involve the entire diaphragm. The eventrated portion of the diaphragm moves paradoxically, just like a paralyzed diaphragm, at fluoroscopy. Eventration is a manifestation of the aging process and generally occurs in older patients; portions of the diaphragm appear to "wear out" as these patient age.

Intraabdominal Process

Organomegaly. The most common intraabdominal process to elevate one diaphragm is organomegaly (usually of the spleen on the left side and the liver on the right). Occasionally, a distended stomach or colon is seen beneath an elevated diaphragm, but this is usually is a secondary phenomenon and does not cause diaphragmatic elevation. In these patients, the elevation usually results from some other cause, such as eventration or paralysis.

Subphrenic Abscess. Subphrenic abscess also causes diaphragmatic elevation because of splinting. Fluoroscopic findings include a diaphragm that moves

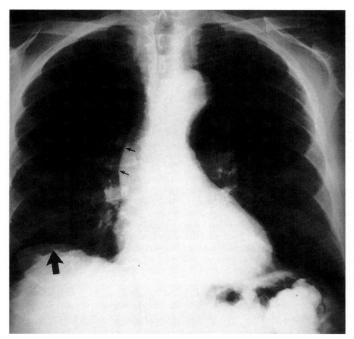

Figure 9.1. Eventration of the diaphragm. A focal bulge from an eventration (*arrows*) can be seen in the right hemidiaphragm. This patient also had a dilated ascending aorta (*small arrows*) from aortic stenosis.

117

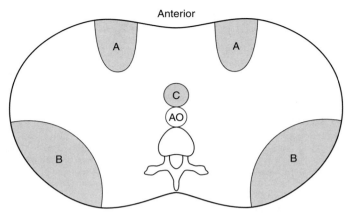

Anterior

Figure 9.2. Axial views of the diaphragmatic foramina. Hernias generally occur through one of these foramina. **A.** Foramina of Morgagni. **B.** Foramina of Bochdalek. **C.** Esophageal foramen.

very poorly or is fixed totally and does not move at all. Subphrenic abscess usually is associated with pleural effusion and atelectasis in the ipsilateral lung.

Subpulmonic Effusion

Though subpulmonic effusion does not cause diaphragmatic elevation, the diaphragm appears to be elevated because the inferior surface of the lung (usually a marker of the diaphragm) is elevated. A measurable distance between the stomach bubble and inferior surface of the lung is suggestive of a subpulmonic effusion on the left side (see Fig. 8.3). A blunted posterior costophrenic sulcus (usually an accompaniment of subpulmonic fluid collection) is suggestive of a subpulmonic effusion on either side. The pleural effusion is readily demonstrated on a decubitus film.

Figure 9.2 shows the diaphragmatic foramina, which is a common place for hernias of the diaphragm. The paired foramina of Morgagni are anterior and medial. Left-sided Morgagni hernias rarely occur, however, because of the presence of the heart, but right-sided Morgagni hernias are relatively common. Both types of hernias generally contain omentum but may contain colon as well.

The paired posterolateral foramina of Bochdalek are the site of the large congenital hernias seen in newborns. Adults occasionally exhibit small Bochdalek hernias, however, which usually contain retroperitoneal structures (e.g., kidney).

By far, the esophageal hiatus is the most common foramen involved with diaphragmatic hernias (Fig. 9.3). The hiatal hernia invariably contains a portion of the stomach. Hiatal hernias can be quite large, and they may present in either

Figure 9.3. Hiatal hernia. Posteroanterior (**A**) and lateral (**B**) films show a mass seen through the heart posteroanteriorly and behind the heart laterally (*arrows*). Herniated stomach (*open arrow*) lies within the mass.

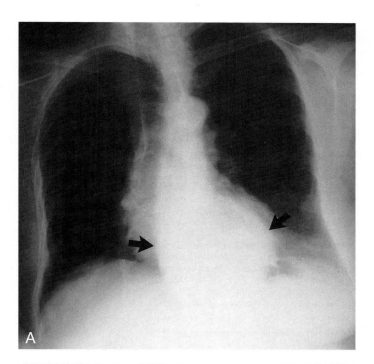

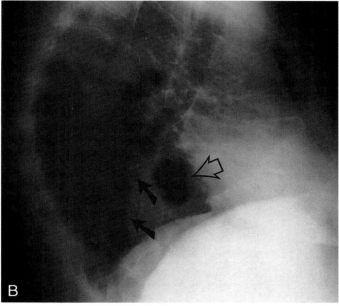

the right or the left hemithorax. When large, they also may contain portions of the colon and even the small bowel. The clue to establishing the diagnosis of a hiatal hernia is that it always has a central location and, even if most of the herniated structures lie in one hemithorax, presents to both sides of the mediastinum.

Fluoroscopy

The simplest, most reliable means for evaluating diaphragmatic motion is direct fluoroscopic observation. Patients are best evaluated in the lateral position. On inspiration, the diaphragm normally moves inferiorly. A paralyzed diaphragm, however, moves superiorly (or paradoxically) during inspiration. A sniff requires rapid downward movement of the diaphragm, and this is the most provocative test of diaphragmatic function. Thus, in some patients, a paralyzed diaphragm may move normally on quiet breathing but paradoxically on sniffing.

Most eventrations of the diaphragm only involve part of the diaphragmatic muscle. Thus, at fluoroscopy, the unaffected portion of the diaphragm is seen to move normally whereas the eventration moves paradoxically. Eventrations may be anterior or posterior. If they involve the entire hemidiaphragm, however, they cannot be differentiated from paralysis. Total eventration of the diaphragm may be the cause for "idiopathic" paralysis of the diaphragm.

Traumatic Rupture

Traumatic rupture of the diaphragm affects patients with blunt abdominal trauma in which a sudden force is exerted on the abdomen and then transmitted to the dome of the diaphragm, thereby tearing the central diaphragmatic tendon. This can occur on either side, but it is more common on the left (Fig. 9.4). It may result in immediate herniation of abdominal contents into the chest at the time of trauma, but 30% to 50% of traumatic hernias are recognized at a later time (often many years after the trauma). The hernia may resemble an elevated hemidiaphragm, but the apparent diaphragm usually is irregular in contour. The hernia contents generally are stomach, colon, or both. A chronic traumatic hernia may be accompanied by a pleural effusion, which often is an ominous sign that indicates strangulation of the hernia.

Tumors

Tumors of the diaphragm are very rare, but occasionally, one encounters a diaphragmatic sarcoma. This sarcoma usually presents as a focal mass in the diaphragm, and on a plain film, it may be impossible to differentiate from an eventration. Magnetic resonance imaging is optimal for evaluating diaphragmatic masses. Some pleural tumors, particularly large pleural fibromas, may simulate a diaphragmatic tumor or an elevated hemidiaphragm.

THE CHEST WALL

Chest wall masses are marked by the extrapleural sign. When seen in profile, an extrapleural mass has a smooth border, because it is covered by parietal pleura. It has its greatest diameter at the midportion of the lesion, and because the parietal pleura is stripped or elevated from the chest wall, the extrapleural mass has acute angles with the chest wall (Fig. 9.5). Pleural tumors may have exactly the

Diaphragm and Chest Wall

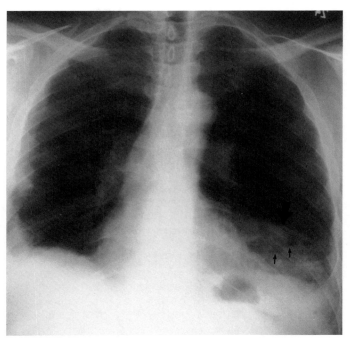

Figure 9.4. Traumatic rupture of the left diaphragm. This 40-year-old man had a density along the left side of the heart (*arrow*) and several air-fluid levels (*small arrows*). These findings should make one suspect herniated bowel into the chest. Note also the old pleural thickening on the right secondary to an old hemothorax.

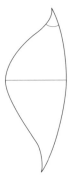

Figure 9.5. The extrapleural sign. Extrapleural masses, when seen in profile, have the greatest diameter at the midportion of the lesion. They also tend to make an acute angle with the chest wall and to have a very smooth profile.

Diaphragm and Chest Wall

same appearance; however, most chest wall lesions involve the underlying bones (usually the ribs). The chest wall lesion may arise from the rib itself and cause extensive destruction of the rib, or it may invade or erode the rib as it arises in the soft tissues adjacent to that rib. The character of the bony involvement generally is suggestive of the nature of the chest wall lesion. A very destructive process in the bone is indicative of a metastatic tumor or an aggressive bone or soft-tissue sarcoma. Erosion of the rib usually is suggestive of a more benign process, such as some form of neurogenic tumor. By far, metastatic tumor to a rib is the most common cause of extrapleural mass (Fig. 9.6).

Rib Lesions

Lesions arising from a rib, whether metastases or primary bone tumors, rarely if ever invade the adjacent ribs. Therefore, a single mass involving two or more adjacent ribs is suggestive of a soft-tissue or lung lesion invading the ribs and not of a primary rib problem.

After metastatic tumor, myeloma and lymphoma are the most common malignancies involving the ribs. Primary bone tumors such as Ewing's sarcoma,

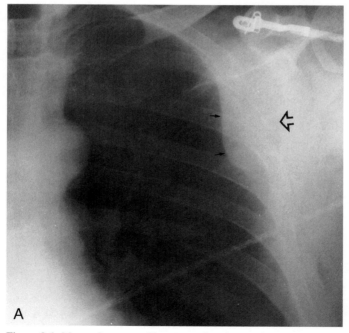

Figure 9.6. Metastatic tumor with an extrapleural mass. **A.** An extrapleural mass in the left upper lung field (*arrows*) with destruction of the left third rib (*open arrow*) by metastatic carcinoma from the right lung. **B.** A similar extrapleural mass (*closed arrows*) with destruction of the right ninth posterior rib (*open arrow*) by metastatic carcinoma from the kidney.

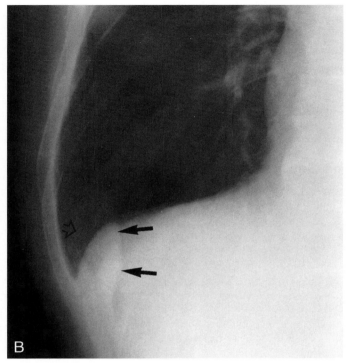

Figure 9.6. (*continued*)

osteosarcoma, and chondrosarcoma also can originate in the ribs or sternum. Benign bony lesions also may cause an extrapleural mass. Osteochondromas are fairly common in ribs, either as solitary lesions or as multiple hereditary osteochondromas. In general, the appearance of benign rib lesions on the chest x-ray is sufficiently characteristic to establish a specific diagnosis.

Causes of Extrapleural Masses

Healing fractures frequently can produce an extrapleural mass and may simulate a metastatic tumor. Fractures of several adjacent ribs in a line are strongly suggestive of trauma as the cause of the fractures. Benign rib lesions usually involve the ribs without development of an extrapleural mass. This is particularly true of bone islands, which often simulate pulmonary nodules and are a common finding on the chest x-ray. Enchondromas also may occur without an extrapleural mass.

Neoplasms are the common cause for extrapleural masses, but infection also occasionally causes a chest wall mass. For example, osteomyelitis may involve the chest wall. Tuberculosis, some fungal infections, and actinomycosis also

123

rarely may involve the chest wall and rib and can create an extrapleural sign (Fig. 9.7).

Neurogenic Tumors

Neurogenic tumors are the most common benign lesion of the chest wall (Fig. 9.8). They usually erode adjacent ribs and create small to large extrapleural masses, and occasionally, they may create rib notching without an apparent soft-tissue mass. These neural tumors usually are ganglioneuromas or schwannomas but sometimes can be a more malignant variety. They usually arise from the intercostal nerves. In addition to being common tumors of the chest wall, neurogenic tumors are the most common posterior mediastinal tumors. Even so,

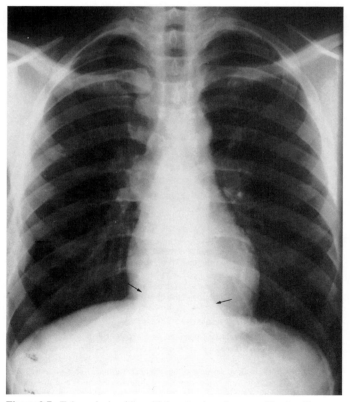

Figure 9.7. Tuberculosis with multiple extrapleural masses. Chest wall masses can be seen protruding in the lung in the right lateral chest wall and in the paraspinal location (*arrows*). These changes resulted from bony (chest wall) tuberculosis in this 27-year-old male drug abuser.

Diaphragm and Chest Wall

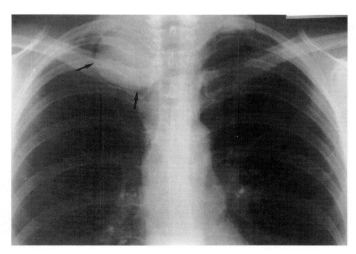

Figure 9.8. Neurogenic tumor. A well-circumscribed mass at the right apex (*arrows*) that resulted from a schwannoma in a 43-year-old woman.

it may be difficult to determine whether a neurogenic tumor arises in the posterior chest wall or the posterior mediastinum. This distinction makes little difference in the differential diagnosis, however, because a tumor in either location likely is a neurogenic tumor.

SUGGESTED READINGS

Alexander C. Diaphragm movements and the diagnosis of diaphragmatic paralysis. Clin Radiol 1966;17:79–87.

Felson B. The extrapleural space. In: Felson B, ed. Chest roentgenology. Philadelphia: WB Saunders, 1973:380–388.

Miller WT, Talman EA. Subphrenic abscess. AJR 1967;101:961–969.

Omell GH, Anderson LS, Bramson RT. Chest wall tumors. Radiol Clin North Am 1973;11:197–215.

Whittaker LD Jr, Lynn HB, Dawson B, Chaves E. Hernias of the foramen of Bochdalek in children. Mayo Clin Proc 1968;43:580–586.

Mediastinum 10

ANATOMIC DIVISIONS

Anatomists have divided the mediastinum into the anterior, middle, and posterior mediastinum, with superior and inferior divisions as well. When evaluating chest films, however, the superior and inferior mediastinal divisions are not useful. The anatomic divisions of the mediastinum are as follows (Fig. 10.1):

1. The posterior border of the anterior mediastinum runs anterior to the great vessels, along the ascending aorta, and anterosuperior to the heart.
2. The posterior border of the middle mediastinum runs posterior to the esophagus to the level of the hilum. It then runs inferior to the hilum and along the posterior margin of the heart to the inferior vena cava.
3. The posterior mediastinum lies posterior to the middle mediastinum and extends to the posterior chest wall.

It certainly is proper to use the anatomic divisions of the mediastinum. For radiologists, however, these divisions are not ideal, because they place certain structures, such as the aorta and the esophagus, in the middle compartment of the upper mediastinum and in the posterior compartment of the lower mediastinum.

To unify the various mediastinal lesions, most radiologists use a slight variation of mediastinal divisions. In this variation, the posterior border of the middle compartment is displaced posteriorly in its inferior portion, so that it lies posterior to the esophagus and anterior to the spine for the length of the mediastinum (Fig. 10.1). This places all of the viscera in the middle compartment, which then can be called the visceral compartment. The posterior compartment also becomes the paraspinal compartment, and it contains only the spine and masses that arise in the paraspinal area.

Mediastinal masses are fairly characteristic in their appearance, and they are fairly constant regarding the compartments in which they occur. Occasionally, a neurogenic tumor occurs in a middle compartment or a cyst in the posterior compartment, but each mediastinal lesion tends to occur in one particular compartment. Thus, the ability to recognize compartment boundaries and knowledge of particular lesions occur in which compartments are very useful.

Many lesions occur more frequently in certain age groups; therefore, the age of the patient may be useful as well. This relationship is less constant than the location of the lesions, however.

Common Anterior Mediastinal Masses

Common anterior mediastinal masses include:

1. Thyroid masses.
2. Thymoma and other thymic masses.
3. Teratoma and germ cell neoplasms.
4. Lymphadenopathy.

Thyroid Masses

Goiter is a very common thyroid mass, and it often displaces the trachea in the neck (Fig. 10.2). As the goiter enlarges, it frequently extends into the upper mediastinum. Thus, the key to a radiographic diagnosis of goiter is recognizing a long, smooth displacement of the trachea, usually to the right or left but sometimes posteriorly and occasionally anteriorly. Thyroid masses generally are con-

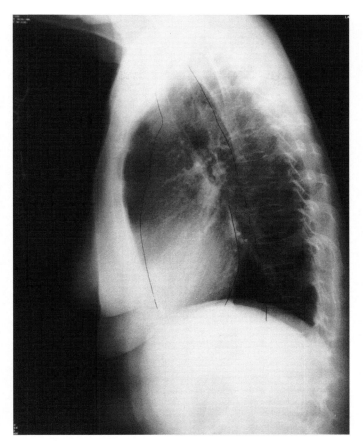

Figure 10.1. Divisions of the mediastinum. The anatomic division into ante-rior, middle, and posterior mediastinum is indicated by the solid lines. The ra-diologic variation of the middle and posterior compartments is indicated by the dotted line.

sidered to arise in the anterior mediastinum, but they also are common in the middle compartment. This is because they grow beside or behind the trachea, which is a visceral compartmental structure.

Other thyroid masses, such as thyroid adenoma or carcinoma, also may extend into the upper mediastinum and displace the trachea. Occasionally, thyroid car-cinoma even may invade the trachea and, on the chest film, cause an irregular stricture of the trachea air column. There is no other way to distinguish benign from malignant thyroid masses on the chest film. All thyroid masses occasion-ally may calcify as well.

Mediastinum

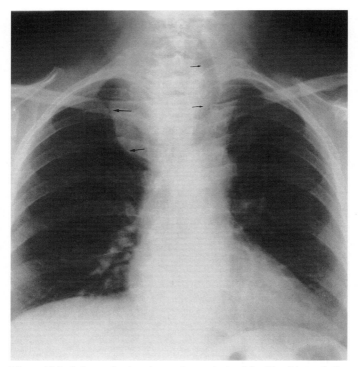

Figure 10.2. Substernal goiter. A mass is seen in the right side of the neck displacing the trachea to the left and extending substernally on the right (*arrows*). This is characteristic of a substernal goiter.

Thymoma and Other Thymic Masses

The normal thymus, some fat, and a few lymph nodes are the only normal inhabitants of the anterior mediastinum. Thymic tumors are one of the more common anterior mediastinal masses. They can occur in any age group but commonly are not seen in those younger than 20 years. They are most common in middle-aged patients (40–60 years).

Thymomas often are associated with paraneoplastic syndromes. The most common of these syndromes is myasthenia gravis, which occurs in 40% of patients with thymoma. (Fifteen percent of patients with myasthenia gravis have a thymoma; many of the others have thymic hyperplasia.) Many other paraneoplastic syndromes have been linked with thymoma, but after myasthenia gravis, the two most common are red cell aplasia and hypogammaglobulinemia. Cushing's syndrome is frequently seen in patients with thymic carcinoids.

Noninvasive thymomas are completely encapsulated histopathologically. When these thymomas are surgically resected, patients are cured of further disease. Invasive thymomas invade the tumor capsule, either microscopically or macroscopically, and subsequently metastasize. Noninvasive or microscopically invasive thymomas appear as well-defined, round or oval anterior mediastinal masses, and one cannot be distinguished from the other (Fig. 10.3). Macroscopic invasion appears as a lobulated or diffusely infiltrating mass (Fig. 10.4).

Thymomas metastasize to the pleura on either side (Fig. 10.4), usually without an associated pleural effusion. Thymic metastases are slow-growing and usually quite amenable to resection, radiation therapy, or chemotherapy. Long survival times are seen in patients with metastatic thymoma.

Calcification occurs in 5% to 10% of patients with thymomas (Fig. 10.3). Calcification also occur in patients with thymic cysts.

Thymolipoma and thymic cysts are other well-encapsulated thymic masses. Thymolipoma frequently is quite large, and it may change its appearance on decubitus films. This is because the large amount of fat in the mass makes it a soft, compliant lesion. Thymic cysts may be suspected from the plain film because of their very round silhouette.

Less common malignant tumors of the thymus are indistinguishable from thymoma. Thymic carcinoids and thymic lymphoma usually are well-encapsulated but sometimes can spread beyond the thymus. Thymic carcinoma, which is a relatively rare tumor, usually spreads in an extracapsular fashion.

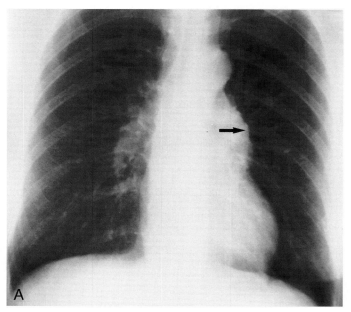

Figure 10.3. Thymoma. **A.** Posteroanterior film shows a mass in the area of the aortopulmonary window (*arrow*) in this 52-year-old woman. **B.** Lateral film of the same woman. The mass, which pvoved to be a benign thymoma, can be faintly seen in the anterior mediastinum (*arrow*). A small amount of calcification is present within it (*small arrows*).

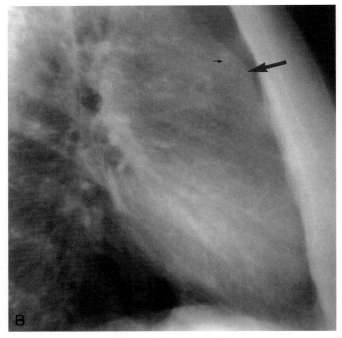

Figure 10.3. *(continued)*

Teratomas and Germ Cell Neoplasms

Mediastinal teratomas are the most common mediastinal germ cell tumor. Radiographically, they usually cannot be distinguished from a thymoma. They frequently are partially calcified, but so are thymomas. Radiographically identifiable fat or teeth are rare in mediastinal teratomas, unlike in abdominal teratomas.

Like thymomas, teratomas may be well-encapsulated and likely are benign, or they may be diffusely spread throughout the anterior mediastinum and definitely malignant (Fig. 10.5). Other germ cell neoplasms such as seminoma, choriocarcinoma, and embryonal cell carcinoma may be primary in the mediastinum. When such a mediastinal germ cell neoplasm is discovered, a primary tumor in the testes or ovary must always be excluded.

Lymphadenopathy

Lymphadenopathy is the most common middle mediastinal mass. In addition, it is common in the anterior mediastinum, though it may not be isolated to the anterior mediastinum. When it is isolated to the anterior mediastinum, lymphadenopathy is strongly suggestive of tumor (most commonly lymphoma but occasionally metastatic tumor). Lymphoma may be indistinguishable from ma-

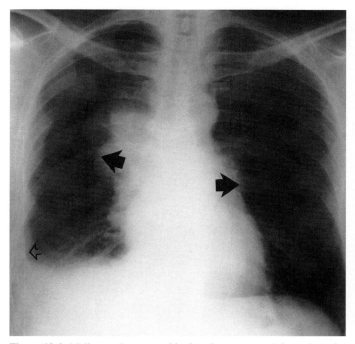

Figure 10.4. Malignant thymoma with pleural metastases. A large, irregular mass can be seen presenting to both sides of the mediastinum (*closed arrows*). Pleural nodules and a right pleural effusion also can be seen (*open arrow*). The mass and nodule findings are characteristic of a malignant thymoma, and the pleural metastases are in keeping with this diagnosis.

lignant thymoma on plain films and computed tomographic (CT) scans (Fig. 10.6). Both types of image show a large mass spreading throughout the anterior mediastinum. Lymphoma also may involve the middle mediastinal nodes, but it is not unusual for it to be isolated to the anterior mediastinum, thereby displacing the vascular structures posteriorly. In patients with a neoplasm having this appearance, lymphoma can be differentiated from malignant thymoma or malignant teratoma only at biopsy.

Effects of Excessive Mediastinal Fat

Excessive mediastinal fat may cause diffuse widening of the mediastinum. This excessive fat generally occurs in the anterior mediastinum, where it widens the mediastinum in a smooth, symmetrical fashion and generally can be recognized as fat. Fat also may occur in the paraspinal area, however, and cause masses around the thoracic spine.

Excessive mediastinal mass generally results from obesity, but it also may result from exogenous steroids.

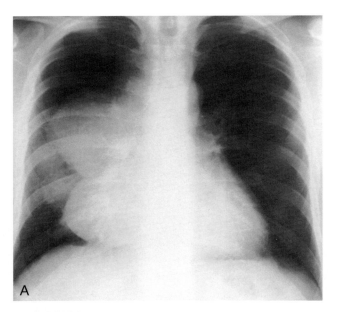

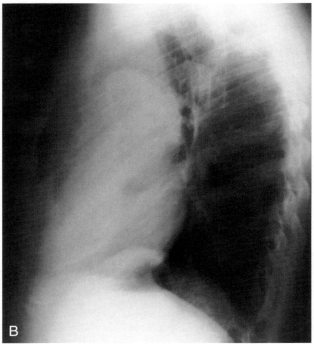

132

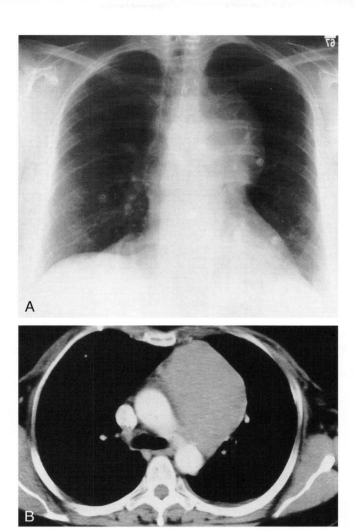

Figure 10.6. Lymphoma involving the anterior mediastinum. The posteroanterior film (**A**) shows a large mediastinal mass. The CT scan (**B**) and MR image (**C**) show that the mass is confined to the anterior mediastinum. This mass might have been a thymoma or teratoma, but it proved to be a non-Hodgkin's lymphoma confined to the anterior mediastinum.

Figure 10.5. Malignant teratoma. **A.** Posteroanterior film. An irregular mass is seen presenting to the right of the mediastinum. **B.** Lateral film. The mass lies in the anterior mediastinum and projects posteriorly. This mass is a malignant teratoma, but it cannot be distinguished radiographically from a malignant thymoma or lymphoma.

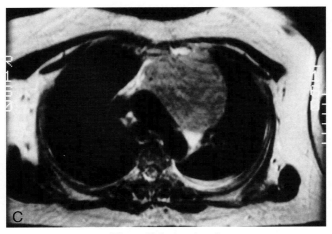

Figure 10.6. (*continued*)

Common Middle Compartmental Masses

Using the radiographic division of the mediastinum, the middle compartment contains all of the viscera except the thymus. Thus, any mass that occurs in the middle compartment can be related to a particular viscus.

The more common middle compartmental masses include:

1. Adenopathy.
   A. Lymphoma.
   B. Metastatic tumor.
   C. Sarcoidosis.
   D. Primary tuberculosis.
   E. Fungal infections.
   F. Human immundeficiency virus (HIV) infection.
   G. Less common causes.
2. Duplication cysts
   A. Mediastinal.
   B. Bronchogenic and esophageal.
   C. Pericardial.
3. Dilated esophagus and esophageal masses.
   A. Benign or malignant tumor.
   B. Esophageal diverticulum.
   C. Dilated esophagus.
4. Lesions of the aorta and great vessels.
   A. Aneurysms.
   B. Venous anomalies.
   C. Tortuous vessels.
   D. Aortic anomalies.
5. Hiatal hernia.
6. Thyroid masses.

Adenopathy

Lymphoma.   Lymphadenopathy is the most common middle mediastinal mass, and metastatic tumor is the most common cause of lymphadenopathy. Bronchogenic carcinoma (with metastases to one hilum, various portions of the mediastinum, or both) is the most common tumor to metastasize to the mediastinum. Tumors from remote locations such as the testes, breast, and kidney as well as melanoma, however, also occasionally metastasize to the mediastinum. In fact, any tumor may do the same on rare occasions.

Lymphoma is another common cause of mediastinal adenopathy (Fig. 10.7). Both Hodgkin's lymphoma and non-Hodgkin's lymphoma usually involve the middle mediastinum but also may concomitantly or solely involve the mediastinum anterior.

Metastatic Tumor.   The appearance of metastatic lymph nodes in the mediastinum varies depending on the location of the nodes. One or multiple node-bearing areas may be involved. Unilateral hilar metastases are common with any tumor but particularly with carcinoma of the lung. Azygos adenopathy and right paratracheal adenopathy are easily identified by thickening of the right tracheal shadow, which normally is only 3- or 4-mm thick. When paratracheal lymphadenopathy is present, however, this stripe may be several centimeters wide.

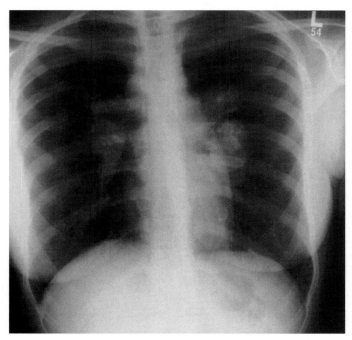

Figure 10.7. Hodgkin's lymphoma of the middle mediastinum resembling sarcoidosis. This 32-year-old woman had bilateral hilar and right paratracheal adenopathy, which is characteristic of sarcoid. In this patient, however, the configuration proved to be non-Hodgkin's lymphoma.

135

Involvement of both hila is rare in patients with bronchogenic carcinoma and uncommon in patients with other tumors. Such involvement is more common in patients with lymphoma (Fig. 10.7) and metastases from a distant site, but it usually is caused by inflammatory lesions.

Sarcoidosis.   Sarcoidosis typically involves the right paratracheal area and both hilar areas (i.e., the "one, two, three sign") (Fig. 10.7). Unlike hilar adenopathy from tumor, however, the hilar adenopathy from sarcoidosis is somewhat more peripheral, involving the peribronchial lymph nodes. These affected lymph nodes have been called "potato" nodes, because they resemble a newly dug cluster of potatoes.

Primary Tuberculosis.   Hilar and mediastinal lymphadenopathy is a frequent manifestation of primary tuberculosis (Fig. 10.8). The hilar adenopathy in patients usually is unilateral, though it can be bilateral.

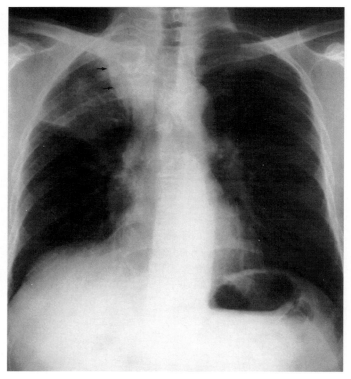

Figure 10.8. Primary tuberculosis with mediastinal adenopathy. This 70-year-old man had patchy atelectasis of the right upper lobe and right paratracheal adenopathy (*arrows*). This appearance is strongly suggestive of primary lung carcinoma but resulted from primary tuberculosis.

Fungal Infections.   Fungal infections also may cause middle mediastinal adenopathy. Histoplasmosis is probably the most common fungal infection to do so, but coccidioidomycosis and blastomycosis may cause hilar and mediastinal lymphadenopathy. Histoplasmosis occasionally is complicated by development of fibrosing mediastinitis, which may be idiopathic but usually is a complication of histoplasmosis. Fibrosing mediastinitis is a noninfectious immune reaction to histoplasma antigens. It causes a fullness of the mediastinum that resembles mediastinal adenopathy and tends to constrict and invade the mediastinal structures, most frequently the superior vena cava, but also the pulmonary artery and veins, occasionally the main stem bronchi, and even the aorta.

HIV Infection.   In patients infected with HIV, mediastinal adenopathy usually results from infection. HIV infection alone may cause peripheral adenopathy, but it does not cause radiographically identifiable mediastinal adenopathy. Mediastinal lymphadenopathy is a common manifestation of primary or reactivation tuberculosis in patients with AIDS. Atypical mycobacteria, which usually do not cause lymphadenopathy in normal hosts, also may present as mediastinal adenopathy in patients with HIV infection. Fungal infections such as coccidioidomycosis, histoplasmosis, and cryptococcus also may cause mediastinal adenopathy in these patients, and rarely, lymphoma or Kaposi's sarcoma produces mediastinal adenopathy in this group. Despite this broad differential diagnosis, mycobacterial diseases remain the most common cause of mediastinal adenopathy in patients with HIV infection.

Less Common Causes.   Silicosis and coal worker's pneumoconiosis are rare causes of mediastinal adenopathy. Silicosis is becoming less common today, but adenopathy is not an uncommon feature of this disease. Berylliosis also occasionally may cause lymphadenopathy. Angioimmunoblastic lymphadenopathy and Casselman's disease are rare causes of mediastinal adenopathy.

Duplication Cysts

Mediastinal.   Duplication cysts of the mediastinum can arise from a bronchogenic origin (i.e., trachea or main stem bronchi) or from an esophageal origin.

Bronchogenic and Esophageal.   Bronchogenic and esophageal duplication cysts are well-circumscribed and tend to occur in characteristic locations. They are filled with fluid and almost never communicate with the esophagus or trachea. The fluid often is quite proteinaceous, and it may have a CT attenuation greater than the normal range for simple fluids, thereby suggesting a solid mass. Bronchogenic cysts usually are subcarinal in location; esophageal cysts tend to be adjacent to the distal esophagus. Even so, these duplication cysts can occur at any location throughout the mediastinum (Fig. 10.9) and even within the lung parenchyma. CT scans may show their cystic nature, but these scans often show attenuations of greater than 20 Hounsfield units. Therefore, the cysts may be confused with solid lesions. Ultrasonography and magnetic resonance (MR) imaging, however, can show their cystic nature.

Pericardial.   Pericardial cysts generally occur at the cardiophrenic angles on either side of the heart (Fig. 10.10). Because the pericardium extends from the aortic arch to the diaphragm, however, pericardial cysts may be seen over a wide range of middle mediastinal locations. These cysts occasionally may communicate with the pericardium, and they may enlarge or decrease in size secondary to an increase or decrease in pericardial effusion. Foramen of Morgagni

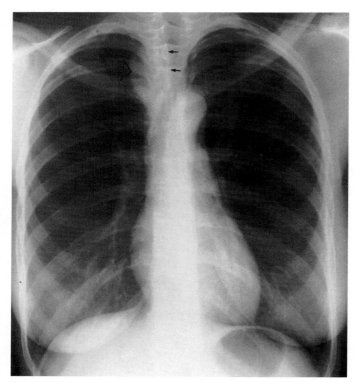

Figure 10.9. Bronchogenic cyst. A bronchogenic cyst is seen in the right upper mediastinum displacing the trachea to the left (*arrows*). This appearance resembles that of a substernal goiter.

hernias and a large pericardial fat pad may resemble pericardial cysts because of their location in the cardiophrenic angles. Cardiophrenic angle masses are almost always benign, though a thymoma rarely may present in this location.

Dilated Esophagus and Esophageal Masses

Dilated Esophagus. A dilated esophagus may have the appearance of a mass in the middle mediastinum (Fig. 10.11). This most commonly is seen among patients with achalasia, but a dilated esophagus occasionally can be seen above a benign stricture of the esophagus—and rarely above a malignant tumor of the

———————————————————————————————————→

Figure 10.11. Achalasia. **A.** Posteroanterior film. The dilated esophagus is seen as a large mass along the right side of the mediastinum (*arrows*). The mass contains air mixed with semisolid material. **B.** Lateral film. The mass lies behind the trachea and the heart and displaces the trachea anteriorly (*arrows*).

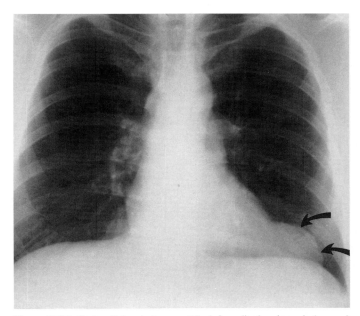

Figure 10.10. Pericardial cyst. A mass at the left cardiophrenic angle (*arrows*) is in a location characteristic for a pericardial cyst. The diagnosis was confirmed at CT.

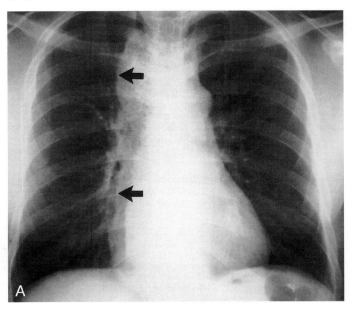

A

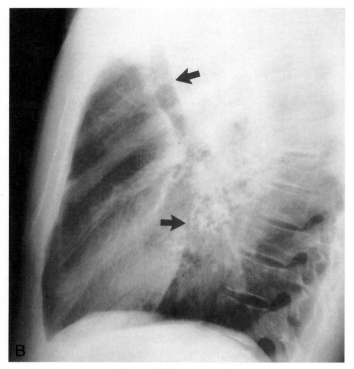

Figure 10.11. (*continued*)

esophagus. A dilated esophagus usually can be suspected on the basis of the elongated contour of the mass. Generally, the mass (i.e., the esophagus) is seen on the right side of the mediastinum, and an air-fluid level often is identified within it. The dilated esophagus also invariably displaces the trachea anteriorly, which can be suggestive that suspected mediastinal mass is actually a dilated esophagus.

Esophageal Diverticulum.   Esophageal diverticula also occasionally can present as a mediastinal mass. This is particularly true of Zenker's diverticulum, which may extend downward from the neck and displace the trachea anteriorly. Diverticula rarely are encountered as masses in other locations, but at times, they may be seen in the epiphrenic area and at the carina.

Benign or Malignant Tumors.   Primary carcinoma of the esophagus generally is symptomatic before the carcinoma becomes large enough to displace the surrounding lung enough to be recognized as a mediastinal mass on the chest film. Tumors of the esophageal wall such as leiomyoma or leiomyosarcoma, however, grow eccentrically in the esophagus, and these tumors may become large enough to be visible on the chest film.

Lesions of the Aorta and Great Vessels

Aneurysms.   Aortic aneurysms may enlarge the aortic contour and present as a mediastinal mass. Saccular aneurysms, which appear as a focal mass, are most common in the area of the aortic arch (Fig. 10.12) but also can occur in the descending aorta. Fusiform enlargement of the aorta can occur secondary to arteriosclerosis or a dissecting aneurysm as well. On a single film of an older patient, it may be impossible to distinguish between a dissecting aneurysm and an arteriosclerotic aneurysm. CT, MR imaging, angiography, or transesophageal echography, however, can make this distinction. If the aortic contour has changed dramatically on plain films obtained in a relatively short period of time (months to several years), a dissection should be suspected.

Venous Anomalies.   Dilatation of the ascending aorta presents to the right side of the mediastinum, and it frequently results from hypertension, arteriosclerosis, or aortic valve disease (see Figs. 4.5 and 12.8). Such dilatation also results,

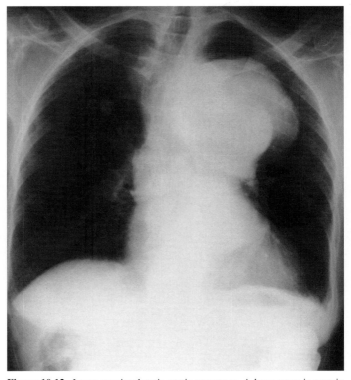

Figure 10.12. Large arteriosclerotic aortic aneurysm. A large mass is seen in the left upper mediastinum, which is inseparable from the aorta and is rather characteristic of an aortic aneurysm. These aneurysms can occur at any level in the thoracic aorta but are most characteristic in the aortic arch.

141

Mediastinum Chapter 10

however, from cystic medial necrosis of the ascending aorta, which commonly occurs in patients with Marfan's syndrome (Fig. 10.13). In young patients with a dilated ascending aorta, this syndrome must be suspected. Syphilitic aortitis may cause dilatation of the ascending aorta as well, but in the United States, tertiary syphilis is extremely rare and syphilitic aortitis occurs only in patients who are very elderly (seventies and eighties).

Tortuous Vessels. Traumatic pseudoaneurysm of the aorta may occur in patients with major trauma, which usually is incurred during a motor vehicle accident. Traumatic pseudoaneurysms generally occur at the ligamentum arteriosus, just distal to the aortic arch, which is the last point of fixation for the thoracic aorta (Fig. 10.14). Traumatic tear of the great vessels may occur as well. In patients who have suffered blunt chest trauma, a widened mediastinum raises the possibility of injury to the aorta or great vessels.

Vascular Anomalies. Anomalies of the aorta and great vessels also may present as mediastinal masses. A right aortic arch occasionally may be mistaken for a mediastinal mass. An aberrant left subclavian artery associated with the right aortic arch almost invariably is also associated with an aortic diverticulum,

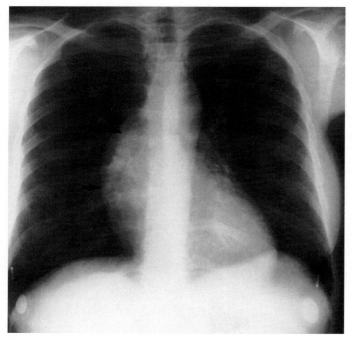

Figure 10.13. Marfan's disease with cystic medial necrosis of the ascending aorta. This 35-year-old woman has a large mass in the right mediastinum at the ascending aorta (*arrows*). The patient's age is suggestive of cystic medial necrosis, and this diagnosis was subsequently confirmed at CT.

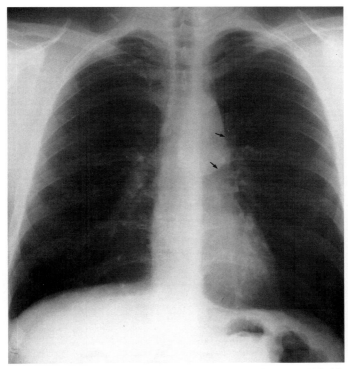

Figure 10.14. Traumatic pseudoaneurysm of the descending aorta. This 32-year-old man had a remote history of a motorcycle accident. The mass in the area of the proximal descending aorta (*arrows*) is characteristic of a traumatic pseudoaneurysm at the area of the ductus.

which may be seen as a mass displacing the trachea anteriorly and projecting to the left side of the mediastinum. An aberrant right subclavian artery sometimes can be associated with an aortic diverticulum as well.

Tortuous great vessels may simulate the appearance of a mediastinal mass, particularly in the upper mediastinum. Occasionally, a venous anomaly such as persistent left superior vena cava also may simulate a mediastinal mass. These entities usually can be suspected on the basis of their elongated appearance.

Hiatal Hernia

Hiatal hernia and goiter generally are not listed as mediastinal masses, but they actually are two of the most common. Hiatal hernia generally can be recognized easily as a hernia that lies posterior to the heart, usually appearing as a round or oval mass seen through the cardiac silhouette (see Fig. 9.3). An air-fluid level often is present within the herniated stomach and provides an important clue to the diagnosis. Occasionally, a hiatal hernia may be quite large, containing colon and even small bowel.

Thyroid Masses

Thyroid masses generally are designated as anterior mediastinal masses, but they often lie beside—or even posterior to—the trachea and are definitely middle mediastinal in location. They are the most common mass behind the trachea in the upper thorax, and the single most common middle mediastinal mass in the upper thorax arises from the thyroid gland (Fig. 10.2). Goiter, thyroid adenoma, thyroid cyst, or thyroid cancer all can displace the trachea to either side and may even displace the trachea anteriorly.

Common Posterior Compartmental Masses

Common masses in the posterior compartment include:

1. Neurogenic tumor.
2. Masses arising from the spine.
   A. Infection.
   B. Neoplasm.
   C. Extramedullary hematopoiesis.

Neurogenic Tumor

The most common mass in the posterior mediastinum is the neurogenic tumor. These masses usually lie in the posterior mediastinal gutter immediately adjacent to the spine, and they may extend through the intervertebral foramen into the spinal canal, where they can displace the spinal cord.

Most posterior compartmental neurogenic tumors are benign and histopathologically are schwannomas, ganglioneuromas, or rarely neurofibromas. In adults, these tumors rarely are malignant, but in infants and children, a posterior mediastinal mass most likely is a neuroblastoma.

Radiographically, a neurogenic tumor usually appears as a round mass adjacent to the spine (Fig. 10.15). It may erode the spine or ribs, or it may expand the intervertebral foramen. Oblique chest films, CT scans, or MR images usually are necessary to show intraspinal extension of the mass (i.e., dumbbell tumor).

The apex of the thorax is a common location for neurogenic tumors. Bilateral apical neurogenic tumors are strongly suggestive of the diagnosis of neurofibromatosis.

Masses Arising from the Spine

Infection. Most cases of thoracic osteomyelitis originate in the bone adjacent to the intervertebral disc and then spread through the disc space, thereby destroying the vertebral end plates. A paraspinal abscess often extends on both sides of the vertebral column at the level of the interspace infection. This is most common among patients in whom tuberculosis involves the thoracic spine (i.e., Pott's disease) but also occurs in those with other infections, including bacterial and fungal infections. In developed countries, bacterial infection is the most common type of spinal infection; in Third World countries, tuberculosis is more

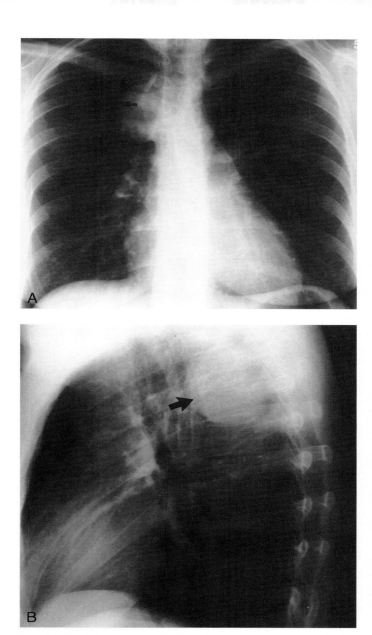

Figure 10.15. Schwannoma. **A.** Posteroanterior film shows a mass extending from the right side of the mediastinum. **B.** Lateral film shows the posterior lo-

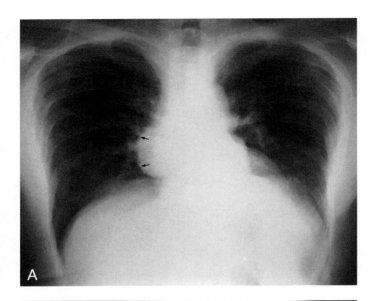

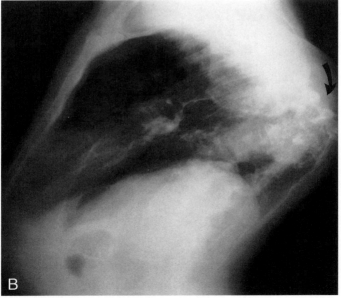

Figure 10.16. Pott's disease with old paraspinal abscess. **A.** Posteroanterior film shows a faintly calcified mass extending from the right side the mediastinum (*arrows*). **B.** Lateral film shows a severe gibbus deformity of the thoracic spine (*arrow*) secondary to previous tuberculosis. The paraspinal mass is a sterile tuberculous abscess.

common. The clue to infection involving the spine is interspace narrowing and destruction of the adjacent vertebral end plates. Occasionally, more than one interspace may be involved as well (Fig. 10.16).

Neoplasm. Primary tumors of the thoracic spine are uncommon, but metastatic tumors are very common. When metastases involve the vertebral bodies, they also may create a paraspinal mass similar to the paraspinal abscess in patients with infection. The destructive process is centered on the vertebral body, however, and the interspace is intact. More commonly, there is destruction of the vertebral bodies without a paraspinal mass, so that a posterior mediastinal mass generally is not seen in patients with metastatic tumor. Primary neoplasms destroy the vertebra in which they arise and may extend into the paraspinal tissue, thereby creating a mass that can be recognized on chest films.

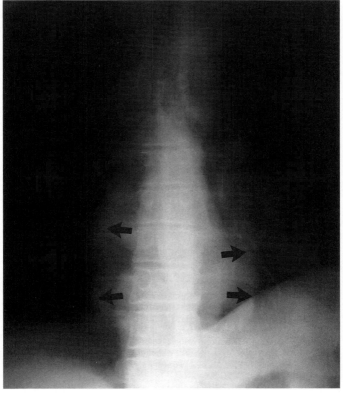

Figure 10.17. Extramedullary hematopoiesis. An overexposed film shows a paraspinal mass extending from both sides of the spine (*arrows*) with no destruction of bone. This proved to be extramedullary hematopoiesis in a patient with spherocytic anemia.

147

Mediastinum

Extramedullary Hematopoiesis. Extramedullary hematopoiesis is an outgrowth of blood-forming elements from the thoracic spine, ribs, or both. It typically occurs in patients with thalassemia, but it also may occur in those with other anemias, such as sickle cell or congenital spherocytic anemia. Extramedullary hematopoiesis may involve any part of the spine, but it generally occurs in the lower thoracic spine (Fig. 10.17). Radiographically, it extends to both sides of the spine, much like a paraspinal abscess; however, there is no evidence of bony destruction as generally seen in patients with a paraspinal abscess.

SUGGESTED READINGS

Arnett EN, Bacos JM, Macher AM, et al. Fibrosing mediastinitis causing pulmonary arterial hypertension, without pulmonary venous hypertension. Clinical and necropsy observations. Am J Med 1977;63:634–641.

Bertelsen S, Malmstrom J, Heerfordt J, Pedersen H. Tumours of the thymic region. Symptomatology, diagnosis, treatment, and prognosis. Thorax 1975;30:19–35.

Christensen EE, Landay MJ, Dietz GW, Brinley G. Buckling of the innominate artery simulating a right apical lung mass. AJR 1978;131:119–124.

Daniel RA, Diveley WL, Edwards WH, Chamberlain N. Mediastinal tumors. Ann Surg 1960;151:783–795.

Davis RD, Oldham HN, Sabiston DC. Primary cysts and neoplasms of the mediastinum: recent changes in clinical presentation, methods of diagnosis, management and results. Ann Thorac Surg 1987;44:229–237.

Egan TJ, Neiman HL, Herman RJ, et al. Computed tomography in the diagnosis of aortic aneurysm dissection of traumatic injury. Radiology 1980;136:141–150.

Goldstein HM, Zornoza J, Hopens T. Intrinsic diseases of the adult esophagus: benign and malignant tumors. Semin Roentgenol 1981;16:183–197.

Godwin JD, Herfkens, KRL, Skioldebrand CG. Evaluation of dissections and aneurysms of the thoracic aorta by conventional and dynamic CT scanning. Radiology 1980;136:125–144.

Goodwin RA, Nickell JA, Des Prez RM. Mediastinal fibrosis complicating healed primary histoplasmosis and tuberculosis. Medicine 1972;51:227–236.

Heitzman ER. The mediastinum. 2nd ed. St. Louis: CV Mosby, 1977:2–24.

Herlitzka AJ, Gale JW. Tumors and cysts of the mediastinum. AMA Arch Surg 1958;76:697–706.

Lyons HA, Calvy GL, Sammons BP. The diagnosis and classification of mediastinal masses. I. A study of 782 cases. Ann Intern Med 1959;51:897–932.

McLoughlin MJ, Weisbrod G, Wise DJ, Yeung HP. Computed tomography in congenital anomalies of the aortic arch and great vessels. Radiology 1981;138:399–403.

Moore AV, Korobkin M, Powers B, et al. Thymoma detection by mediastinal CT: patients with myasthenia gravis. AJR 1982;138:217–223.

Proto AV. Mediastinal anatomy: emphasis on conventional images with anatomic and computed tomographic correlations. J Thorac Imag 1987;2:1–48.

Reed JC, Hallett KK, Feigin DS. Neural tumors of the thorax: subject review from the AFIP. Radiology 1978;126:9–17.

Rietz KA, Werner B. Intrathoracic goiter. Acta Chir Scand. 1960;119:379–391.

Rubush JL, Gardner JR, Boyd WC, Ehrenhaft JL. Mediastinal tumors: review of 186 cases. J Thorac Cardiovasc Surg 1973;65:216–222.

Sabiston DC, Scott HW. Primary tumors and cysts of the mediastinum. Ann Surg 1952;136;777–797.

11 Pulmonary Vessels

RADIOGRAPHIC PATTERNS IN PULMONARY AND CARDIAC ABNORMALITIES

Alterations in the normal vascular patterns of the lung may provide considerable information about pulmonary and cardiac abnormalities. The following six patterns aid in establishing the diagnosis of these diseases, particularly cardiac disease:

1. Normal.
2. Cephalized vessels.
3. Diffusely increased vessels.
4. Diffusely decreased vessels.
5. Pruned vessels.
6. Asymmetric vessels.

The pulmonary vessels have a characteristic radiographic pattern. They appear as a series of branching lines that radiate from the hilum. The caliber of these vessels smoothly tapers from the hilum to the periphery of the lung, and the vessels are not apparent radiographically in the 1 to 2 cm of lung adjacent to the chest wall. In upright individuals, gravity causes the lower lobe vessels to be significantly larger than the upper lobe vessels, but in supine individuals, the dorsal vessels are larger than the ventral vessels.

Normal Vessels

Unfortunately, a normal vascular pattern does not exclude physiologic or histopathologic vascular abnormalities. For example, pulmonary embolism is a common clinical problem in which the vascular pattern is usually normal. Similarly, pulmonary vasculitides may have a radiographically normal vascular pattern despite severe histopathologic and physiologic abnormalities. A left-to-right shunt increases blood flow into the pulmonary vessels, but this is not apparent radiographically until the shunt is approximately 3:1. Fortunately, in many instances, alteration of the pulmonary vasculature does occur, which in turn can aid in establishing a clinical diagnosis.

Cephalized Vessels

Cephalization is the reversal of the normal vascular pattern in upright individuals. In these individuals, the upper lobe vessels are larger than the lower lobe vessels (Fig. 11.1). The exact cause of this is debatable, but cephalization is thought to result from spasm of the lower lobe vessels caused by interstitial edema.

Cephalization is well known as a manifestation of left heart failure (see Fig. 12.1), but it does not occur in patients with acute heart failure (e.g., myocardial infarction). Cephalization is a manifestation of chronic left ventricular failure, and patients with chronic left ventricular disease such as ischemic or hypertensive cardiomyopathy show chronic cephalization of their pulmonary vessels. Cephalization becomes more evident when patients are in overt heart failure (see Fig 12.1). If one examines a film obtained before the acute exacerbation, however, it often is apparent that cephalization was present before that exacerbation.

149

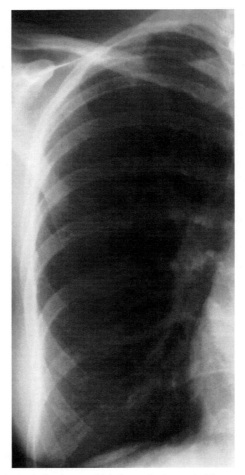

Figure 11.1. Cephalization resulting from mitral senosis. The upper lobe vessels are slightly larger than the lower lobe vessels; the reverse should be true.

Cephalization almost always results from any problem that chronically impedes blood flow into the left heart, and mitral stenosis is a classic cause of cephalization (Fig. 11.1). Cephalization in mitral stenosis frequently is termed *pulmonary venous hypertension*, which is just another name for cephalization. If pulmonary arterial and venous pressures are measured in patients with cephalization, these pressures are chronically mildly elevated. Other causes of obstructed inflow to the heart such as atrial myxoma or pulmonary vein tumor also may cause cephalization.

Pulmonary Vessels

Diffusely Increased Vessels

A diffuse increase in size of the pulmonary vessels usually results from cardiac disease, especially acute left ventricular failure. Left-to-right shunts also cause increased blood flow, which is apparent radiographically as a diffuse increase in pulmonary vessel size (Fig. 11.2; see Fig. 12.10). A 2.5:1 or 3:1 (or even greater) shunt is necessary for observers to perceive the vessels as being enlarged. In a similar fashion, minor degrees of left ventricular failure may not cause radiographically identifiable dilatation of the pulmonary vessels.

Certain lung problems also may cause an *apparent* increase in size of the pulmonary vessels. Patients with chronic bronchitis and some with emphysema may show prominent vessels, a finding which has been designated as the "in-

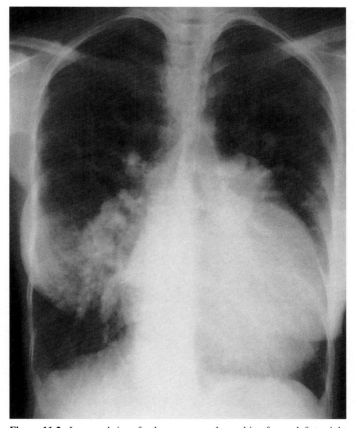

Figure 11.2. Increased size of pulmonary vessels resulting from a left-to-right shunt. This 40-year-old woman had tricuspid atresia, with both right-to-left and left-to-right shunts with enlargement of the pulmonary vessels indicating a dominant left-to-right shunt.

151

Pulmonary Vessels

creased markings pattern." Pulmonary veno-occlusive disease is a rare cause of increased pulmonary vasculature. In patients with known pulmonary hypertension but apparent left heart failure, this diagnosis should be considered.

Diffusely Decreased Vessels

Pulmonary vessels appear to be diffusely decreased in many patients with pulmonary emphysema, and this is accompanied by hyperinflation of the lung fields. The appearance of diminished pulmonary vessels may be quite diffuse, or it may be focal if the pattern of emphysema is heterogeneous. Pulmonary vessels will be absent in the area of bullae.

Some right-to-left shunts (Fig. 11.3) also may result in a radiographically identifiable decrease in pulmonary vascular caliber. This most often results from right-to-left shunts, which have associated pulmonary stenosis (e.g., tetralogy of Fallot).

Pruned Vessels

Pruned vessels refers to the "pruned tree" appearance of the pulmonary vessels in patients with pulmonary hypertension. The central pulmonary arteries are enlarged, and the more peripheral arteries either taper abruptly or are cut off— much like branches of a pruned tree are amputated (Fig. 11.4).

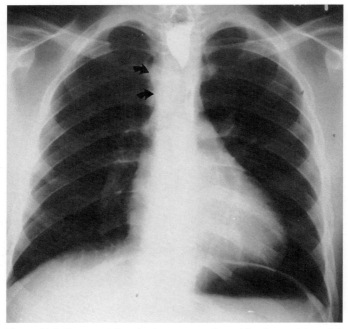

Figure 11.3. Decreased size of pulmonary vessels resulting from a right-to-left shunt in an adult with tetralogy of Fallot. Pulmonary vessels are diffusely decreased, and a right aortic arch is present (*arrows*).

Pulmonary Vessels

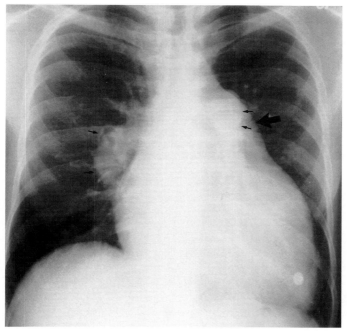

Figure 11.4. Pruned pulmonary vessels resulting from pulmonary hypertension. Large central pulmonary arteries are present (*small arrows*), but the peripheral vessels are small (pruned). There also is enlargment of the heart and considerable enlargement of the main pulmonary artery segment (*large arrow*).

The most common cause of pulmonary hypertension is obstructive lung disease such as emphysema. Pulmonary hypertension also can be seen, however, with restrictive lung diseases such as pulmonary fibrosis or sarcoidosis.

Patients with long-standing left heart failure pass through a stage of cephalization (i.e., pulmonary venous hypertension). Eventually, these patients may reach more severe pulmonary arterial hypertension as well.

Pulmonary hypertension also occurs in some patients with left-to-right shunts. Increased pulmonary vascular resistance reduces the shunt fraction, thereby resulting in pulmonary hypertension. In some patients, pulmonary vascular resistance rises to a point at which the blood flow actually reverses, thus resulting in a right-to-left shunt in someone who previously had a left-to-right shunt (i.e., Eisenmenger's syndrome).

Primary pulmonary hypertension is a disease of unknown cause that produces stenosis or obstruction of pulmonary arteries and resultant pulmonary hypertension. This disease most frequently affects young women. There is no effective therapy other than lung transplantation.

Chronic pulmonary emboli are another cause of pulmonary hypertension. This disease may be recognized on plain films because of the heterogeneity of

Pulmonary Vessels Chapter 11

pulmonary blood flow (i.e., some areas with severely diminished flow and others with increased flow). Pulmonary hypertension also can be caused by certain drugs, such as the diet drugs fen-phen (a combination of fenfluramine and phenteramine and redux [dexfenfluramine]) and the older drug aminorex. It also may be associated with vasculitis secondary to cocaine or with collagen vascular diseases such as lupus erythematosus or scleroderma. In addition, it occasionally may be associated with Wegener's granulomatosis. Pulmonary hypertension also may be caused by portal hypertension.

Asymmetric Vessels

The patterns described thus far in this chapter have been symmetrical. Occasionally, however, vessels can be asymmetrical and indicative of pulmonary parenchymal or pulmonary vascular disease.

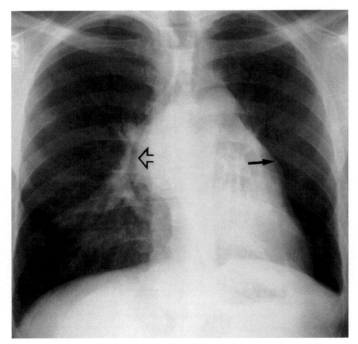

Figure 11.5. Asymmetrical pulmonary vessels resulting from pulmonary artery atresia. This 34-year-old man had asymmetrical vessels, with those on the right being large and those on the left being small. Small vessels can result from pulmonary stenosis, but these are the result of pulmonary atresia with bronchial arteries filling the left pulmonary arteries. This patient also had a small atrial septal defect with a prominent main pulmonary segment (*closed arrow*) and a mediastinal mass (*open arrow*) that later proved to be a bronchogenic cyst.

154

Unilateral diminution in vascular size occurs with several conditions. Occasionally, a large pulmonary embolus may organize in the pulmonary artery and cause a chronic embolus. In such patients, the central pulmonary artery appears to be large and the peripheral vessels diminished. Multiple chronic emboli also may cause asymmetrical vessels but are heterogeneous rather than unilateral in distribution.

Either pulmonary artery may be hypoplastic or even absent. The pulmonary vessels on that side will be small, as will the central pulmonary artery. In patients with pulmonary atresia, the pulmonary arteries in the lung are filled by collateral flow from the bronchial vessels (Fig. 11.5).

Swyer-James syndrome is a complication secondary to a neonatal infection such as bronchiolitis. The involved lung is small, and the pulmonary artery is hypoplastic. The pulmonary vessels are small throughout the lung. The patient also may have extensive bronchiectasis involving that lung (see Fig. 2.6), may have air trapped within the involved lung, or both.

Lung carcinoma sometimes can cause hypoperfusion of the involved lung. Radiation to one lung often will be associated with fibrosis and retraction of the vessels medially, with diminution in size of the remaining vessels. Tuberculosis and sometimes pneumonia can cause hypoplasia of a pulmonary artery with diminished vessels as a sequela of the disease (if unilateral).

Focal asymmetry of the vessels occasionally can occur in patients with acute pulmonary embolus (i.e., Westermark's sign). Most patients with pulmonary emboli have a normal chest film, but a focal asymmetry sometimes can be recognized, particularly if there is a large area of hypoperfusion. Bullae and blebs are other causes of focal asymmetry of the vessels, in which the hyperinflated bulla displaces the normal vessels to one corner of the lung.

SUGGESTED READINGS

Alavi A, Palevsky HI, Weiss DW. Pulmonary hypertension secondary to chronic thromboembolism. J Nucl Med 1990;31:1–9.

Ball KP, Goodwin JF, Harrison CV. Massive thrombotic occlusion of the large pulmonary arteries. Circulation 1956;14:744–766.

Felson B. The hila and pulmonary vessels. In: Felson B, ed. Chest roentgenology. Philadelphia: WB Saunders, 1973;185–210.

Fishman AP. Pulmonary hypertension. In: Wyngarrden J, Smith L, eds. Cecil's textbook of medicine. Philadelphia: WB Saunders, 1988;293–302.

Fleischner FG. Unilateral pulmonary embolism with increased compensatory circulation through the unoccluded lung. Roentgen observations. Radiology 1959;73:591–599.

Heath D, Smith P. Pulmonary vascular disease secondary to lung disease. In: Moser KM, ed. Pulmonary vascular disease. New York: Marcel Dekker, 1979;387–426.

Kerley P. Radiology in heart disease. Br Med J 1933;2:594–627.

Moser KM, Olson LK, Schusselberg M, Daly PO, Dembitsky WP. Chronic thromboembolic occlusion in the adult can mimic pulmonary artery agenesis. Chest 1989;95:503–508.

Sostman HD, Rapaport S, Gottschalk A, Greenspan RH. Imaging of pulmonary embolism. Invest Radiol 1986;21:443–454.

Thurlbeck WM, Simon G. Radiographic appearance of the chest in emphysema. AJR 1978;130:429–440.

Heart **12**

Entire textbooks are written about the heart, and cardiac problems cannot be dealt with here in depth. It would probably be remiss, however, to discuss chest radiology without at least a brief chapter on cardiac problems.

RADIOGRAPHIC PATTERNS IN LEFT VENTRICULAR FAILURE

The most common cardiac problem depicted on chest films involving the heart is left ventricular failure. Characteristically, left ventricular failure passes through several radiographic stages:

> 1. Enlarged pulmonary vessels, with or without cephalization.
> 2. Interstitial pulmonary edema.
> 3. Alveolar edema.
> 4. Pleural effusion.

Enlarged Pulmonary Vessels

Any of the four findings just mentioned can occur with or without cardiomegaly. They usually are accompanied by cardiomegaly, however, with left ventricular enlargement.

The earliest manifestation of left heart failure is enlargement of the pulmonary vasculature. In patients with chronic left heart failure, the vessels frequently are cephalized, and the heart failure manifests mostly with enlargement of the upper lobe vessels (Fig. 12.1). In patients without chronic left heart failure, all of the vessels are enlarged when the patient develops acute left heart failure.

Interstitial Pulmonary Edema

The next phase of left heart failure is transudation of fluid into the interstitium, thereby producing interstitial pulmonary edema (Fig. 12.2). The result is a diffuse increase in the interstitial pulmonary markings, with a linear pattern. Interstitial edema also causes a loss of definition in the pulmonary vessels and bronchi on chest films; this finding is termed *perivascular* or *peribronchial cuffing*.

Alveolar Edema

Many patients proceed rapidly into alveolar pulmonary edema, and the phase of interstitial pulmonary edema is never seen radiographically. Patients with alveolar edema have transudation of interstitial edema into the alveoli, thereby resulting in diffuse alveolar consolidation (Fig. 12.3). Characteristically, this consolidation has a central distribution, with a butterfly or bat-wing pattern, but alveolar edema secondary to cardiac failure can have numerous presentations (see Fig. 1.1). It may be unilateral, particularly if the patient tends to lie on one side, or it may be patchy and somewhat resemble patchy aspiration. It even may be focal and resemble pneumonia.

The clue to the diagnosis of alveolar edema is that the edema changes over time and moves or shifts from one part of the lung to another. Alveolar edema may be impossible to differentiate radiographically from diffuse pulmonary hemorrhage or diffuse infection. Cardiac pulmonary edema also frequently cannot be differentiated radiographically from noncardiac pulmonary edema. Thus, the clinical history and findings are extremely useful for identifying the cause

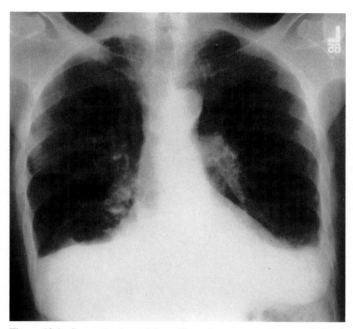

Figure 12.1. Congestive heart failure. The pulmonary vessels are cephalized, with the upper lobe vessels being larger than the lower lobe vessels. Moderate bilateral pleural effusions are present, and the central pulmonary arteries are somewhat enlarged, which is a frequent finding in patients with chronic left heart failure. Bilateral pleural effusions are present as well.

of a diffuse alveolar process. Cardiac failure is one of the more common causes. It also may accompany other alveolar processes, however. Therefor, part of the alveolar consolidation may be caused by noncardiac pulmonary edema, bleeding, or infection, and the cardiac failure may be superimposed and contribute to the alveolar filling. Even chronic processes such as alveolar proteinosis or florid interstitial lung disease may be difficult to differentiate from pulmonary edema without older films or a patient history of chronic lung disease.

Pleural Effusion

Pleural effusion commonly results from heart failure—and almost invariably a combination of left and right heart failure. The pleural effusion may be associated with any of the previously described findings of heart failure (i.e., enlarged pulmonary vessels, interstitial pulmonary edema, or alveolar edema), or it may associated with none of these. Chronic heart failure commonly causes a pleural effusion without other obvious findings of left heart failure. The heart generally is enlarged, but the pleural effusion may be large enough to obscure the cardiac shadow, thereby making the cardiac enlargement difficult to recognize.

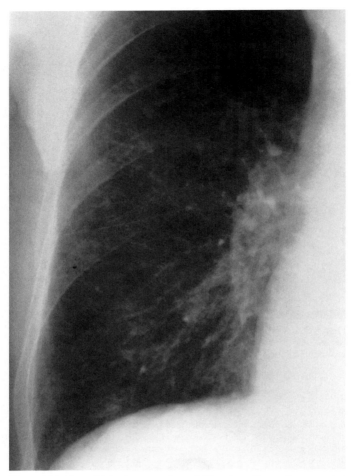

Figure 12.2. Interstitial pulmonary edema. Diffuse lung disease that somewhat resembles interstitial fibrosis is present, but this disease is linear and has multiple Kerley lines. These changes are caused by interstitial pulmonary edema.

Pleural effusion secondary to heart failure must be differentiated from other causes of pleural effusion. This usually is accomplished by the clinician, who identifies a transudative effusion at thoracentesis in a patient with heart failure. Bilateral pleural effusions are suggestive of heart failure. A unilateral effusion may be suggestive of heart failure if it is on the right side, but an isolated left pleural effusion is rare in patients with heart failure.

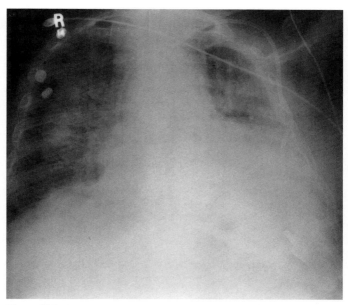

Figure 12.3. Cardiac alveolar edema. Note the diffuse central consolidation of the lungs resulting from alveolar edema secondary to acute congestive heart failure. An absent right shoulder girdle can be incidentally noted as well.

CARDIAC ANATOMY

Figure 12.4 represents the various cardiac structures as seen on posteroanterior and lateral chest films. To understand the location of the various chambers, it is best to visualize them as they would appear on an angiocardiogram. Ultimately, however, one depends on recognizing the border-forming structures.

On the posteroanterior film, the border-forming structures on the right side (moving superiorly) are right atrium, ascending aorta, and superior vena cava. On the left side, they are the left ventricle (rarely the left atrial appendage), main pulmonary artery segment, and aortic knob. The left atrial appendage sometimes projects along the left heart border between the main pulmonary artery and the left ventricular shadow. This occurs almost exclusively in patients with rheumatic heart disease, so it is not a common finding in patients with left atrial enlargement. Most cases of left atrial enlargement have some other cause, usually functional mitral regurgitation or cardiomyopathy (Fig. 12.5).

On the lateral view, the border-forming structures (moving anteriorly from the diaphragm upward) are the right ventricle, occasionally a bit of the main pulmonary artery, and the ascending aorta. Right ventricular enlargement is often difficult to recognize, but it is accompanied almost invariably by enlargement of the main pulmonary artery segment. This is a solid clue that the right

159

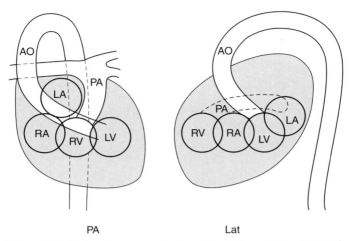

Figure 12.4. The heart on posteroanterior and lateral views. *AO*, aorta; *LA*, left atrium; *LV*, left ventricle; *PA*, pulmonary artery; *RA*, right atrium; *RV*, right ventricle.

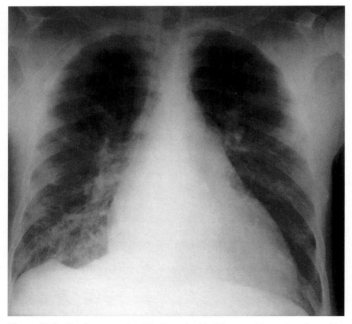

Figure 12.5. Cardiomyopathy. The heart in this 24-year-old man is enlarged in a diffuse fashion, and mild congestive failure is present. This cardiac enlargement was caused by a viral cardiomyopathy.

ventricle probably is enlarged. The right ventricular shadow in normal patients extends for one-third of the retrosternal space, from the diaphragm to the top of the manubrium. In a patient with definite right ventricular enlargement, the right ventricle touches the sternum for one-half of the retrosternal space (or more). Between one-third and one-half extension is equivocal enlargement of the right ventricle. Unfortunately, however, many patients with right ventricular enlargement fall in this category.

Posterior border-forming structures (moving from the diaphragm upward) are the left ventricle and left atrium. Left ventricular enlargement is recognized by the shadow of the left ventricle projecting for 2 cm or more behind the inferior vena cava at a level 2 cm above the junction of the inferior vena cava and the left ventricular shadow. Left atrial enlargement is superior to the left ventricle and displaces the left main stem bronchus posteriorly. Left atrial enlargement also can be seen as a double density through the right side of the heart (Fig. 12.6) and overlying the shadow of the right atrium and the ascending aorta.

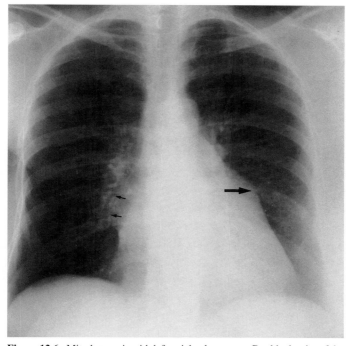

Figure 12.6. Mitral stenosis with left atrial enlargement. Double density of the left atrium is seen projecting from the right side of the heart (*small arrows*). Enlargement of the main pulmonary artery and left atrial appendage (*large arrow*) are seen as well.

Heart

ACQUIRED HEART DISEASE

The most common cardiac diseases depicted on plain chest films are acquired heart diseases, which usually enlarge the left ventricle or all of the cardiac chambers. Hypertension, cardiac ischemia, and cardiomyopathy (Fig. 12.5) are examples of such diseases. Diffuse enlargement of the heart cannot be distinguished from pericardial effusion, however, which may have exactly the same appearance. Usually, patients with pericardial effusions do not have accompanying heart failure, but this also may be true of patients with cardiomyopathy. Cardiac echography is the usual way of recognizing pericardial effusion. A few subtle radiographic signs, such as displaced epicardial fat on the lateral film (Fig. 12.7), can be used as well, however, these seldom are present in patients with pericardial effusion.

Another common acquired heart disease is pulmonary hypertension secondary to pulmonary, cardiac, or vascular problems. In patients with pulmonary hypertension, the right ventricle is enlarged, and the main pulmonary segment

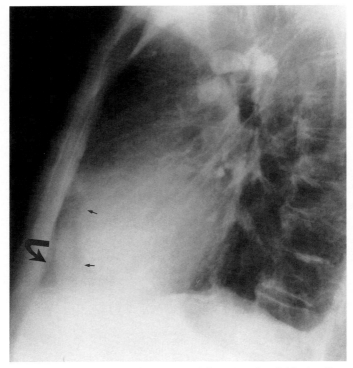

Figure 12.7. Pericardial effusion on a lateral film. The epicardial fat (*small arrows*) is displaced from the pericardial fat (*large arrow*), and between the two is a pericardial effusion.

is almost invariably enlarged as well (see Fig. 11.4). The right atrium also may be enlarged because of functional tricuspid regurgitation.

Left heart failure generally can be recognized on the basis of the radiographic findings mentioned in the previous discussion on heart failure. Right heart failure is a clinical diagnosis, however, and has no good radiographic signs on the chest film. Liver enlargement, ascites, or enlargement of the superior vena cava sometimes can be recognized, but right heart failure generally is better diagnosed on the basis of a physical examination.

Valvular Heart Disease

Valvular heart disease can be congenital, rheumatic, arteriosclerotic, or infectious. (Congenital valvular heart disease is discussed later.)

Rheumatic

Rheumatic heart disease is becoming less and less common. The valve most often involved in rheumatic heart disease is the mitral valve, with either stenosis or insufficiency (Fig. 12.6). The left atrium should be large in both stenosis and insufficiency, but the left ventricle also should be enlarged in insufficiency. The next most common valve involved in rheumatic heart disease is the aortic, with either stenosis or insufficiency. Left ventricular enlargement and enlargement of the ascending aorta are characteristic findings in aortic valvular disease, and tricuspid stenosis, insufficiency, or both result in right atrial enlargement. Rheumatic mitral and aortic valvular disease may occur on an isolated basis. Mitral and aortic valvular disease frequently are combined, however, and tricuspid disease almost is always associated with the other two.

Arteriosclerotic

Aortic stenosis is a fairly common problem in elderly patients because of arteriosclerotic involvement of the aortic valve. Calcification may be seen in the aortic valve on plain films, but the cardiac silhouette usually is normal in size, even in patients with severe or critical aortic stenosis. Calcification commonly occurs in the mitral and aortic annulus in older patients; however, this generally is a benign finding. It may be indistinguishable from valvular calcification.

Infectious

Bacterial infections occasionally involve the cardiac valves (i.e., bacterial endocarditis). When they do, they generally cause insufficiency. The cardiac silhouette may be normal, or there may be enlargement of various cardiac structures (e.g., left ventricle in aortic insufficiency, right atrium in tricuspid insufficiency, left atrium in mitral insufficiency). The valves usually are involved are the aortic valve on the left side of the heart and the tricuspid valve on the right, but any valve can be involved.

CONGENITAL HEART DISEASE

Valvular Lesions

Congenital aortic stenosis or insufficiency is one of the more common congenital valvular heart diseases (Fig. 12.8). These patients characteristically have enlargement of the left ventricle and ascending aorta. On the posteroanterior film,

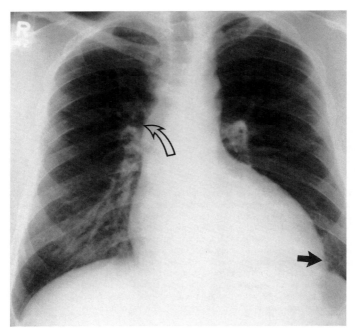

Figure 12.8. Congenital aortic stenosis. The left ventricle (*closed arrow*) and ascending aorta (*open arrow*) are both enlarged in this 27-year-old man with congenital aortic stenosis.

this resembles a "schmoo" (i.e., an animal made famous in Al Capp's comic strip). Mitral stenosis or insufficiency also sometimes occurs, and rarely, the tricuspid valve is displaced inferiorly into the right ventricle, thereby producing inefficient handling of the atrial blood and dilatation of the right atrium (i.e., Ebstein's anomaly) (Fig. 12.9).

Left-to-Right Shunts

There are three common left-to-right shunts: atrial septal defect, ventricular septal defect (VSD), and patent ductus arteriosus (PDA). Of these, atrial septal defect is most likely to continue undetected into adulthood (Fig. 12.10). In adults, VSD is very likely to be complicated by pulmonary hypertension (i.e., Eisenmenger's syndrome) (Fig. 12.11), with reversal of the left-to-right shunt. PDA is unlikely to persist into adulthood, because the ductus usually closes spontaneously. Occasionally, however, a larger ductus can persist and present during adulthood.

Two plain-film findings are indicative of a left-to-right shunt:

1. The vessels should be diffusely increased, and in particular, the central vessels should be enlarged. A shunt of at least 2.5: is necessary to appreciate vascular enlargement.

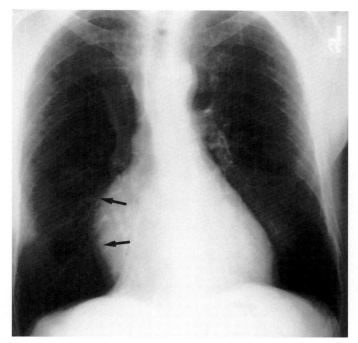

Figure 12.9. Ebstein's anomaly. A dilated right atrium (*arrows*) is seen in this 34-year-old man with Ebstein's anomaly, but the remainder of the heart appears to be normal.

2. The main pulmonary artery segment is be enlarged with any left-to-right shunt.

The key differential findings in the cardiac silhouette of a patient with a left-to-right shunt depends on the alteration of two specific structures: the left atrium, and the aorta. In patients with an atrial septal defect, the left atrium is normal in size, but in patients with a VSD or PDA, the left atrium is enlarged. Think of it this way: in an atrial septal defect, increased blood flow into the left atrium is decompressed through the atrial septal defect into the right atrium. In patients with VSD or PDA, the left atrium must carry at least three times as much blood for every heartbeat, so the atrium must be at least three times larger than normal. Thus, the left atrium should be large in patients with VSD or PDA.

The second structure in which an alteration is useful for the differential diagnosis is the ascending aorta. Using the same analogy as that for the left atrium, the ascending aorta will be enlarged in patients with PDA (because it carries more blood) but normal in size in patients with VSD (because the blood flow through the aorta is normal or even diminished).

Occasionally, a very small, hemodynamically insignificant shunt may occur. In such patients, the cardiac silhouette is normal. In patients with a hemody-

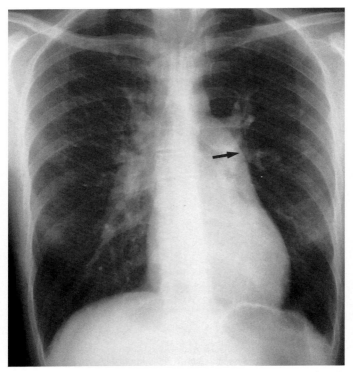

Figure 12.10. Atrial septal defect. Enlarged vessels and an enlarged main pulmonary artery (*arrow*) are present in this 25-year-old asymptomatic woman.

namically insignificant VSD (i.e., maladie de Roger), a loud murmur may be present (because of a small hole in the muscular ventricular septum), but the chest film is normal.

In patients with a prolonged left-to-right shunt in whom pulmonary hypertension has developed, calcification also may develop in the pulmonary arteries (Fig. 12.12). This usually occurs in patients from 30 to 50 years of age. Calcified pulmonary vessels in any patient with pulmonary hypertension, however, is strongly indicative of a preexisting left-to-right shunt with Eisenmenger's physiology as a cause for the pulmonary hypertension. Occasionally, a small amount of focal calcification may occur in the main pulmonary artery of patients with a persistent PDA. Unlike patients with Eisenmenger's syndrome, this calcification usually is very local in the pulmonary artery, and it does not involve all of the pulmonary vessels.

Right-to-Left Shunts (Cyanotic Heart Disease)

The five common right-to-left shunts each begin with a "T":

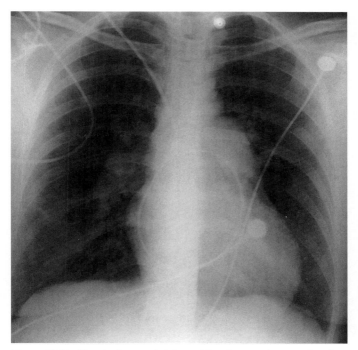

Figure 12.11. Ventricular septal defect with pulmonary hypertension (i.e., Eisenmenger's syndrome). The main pulmonary artery is quite enlarged, and the central pulmonary arteries are pruned bilaterally. These findings are indicative of pulmonary hypertension and could be the result of several possible causes. In this patient, the cause was a ventricular septal defect. The left atrium is not enlarged because of development of the pulmonary hypertension.

1. **Tetralogy of Fallot.**
2. **Transposition.**
3. **Truncus arteriosus.**
4. **Tricuspid atresia.**
5. **Total anomalous pulmonary venous return.**

Patients with any of these shunts should be cyanotic. The most common of these congenital cyanotic lesions is tetralogy of Fallot. Tetralogy of Fallot may persist undetected into adulthood (i.e., pink tet) (Fig. 12.3), and there are several hallmarks of the adult tetralogy:

1. The heart generally is normal in size.
2. The pulmonary blood flow is diminished because of pulmonary stenosis.
3. The cardiac shape is a "boot-shaped" heart (Fig. 12.13). In part, this shape results from right ventricular hypertrophy, which causes an upturned cardiac apex. The shape primarily results from infundibular pulmonary stenosis, which causes a concave or "caved-in" appearance of the left heart border.

167

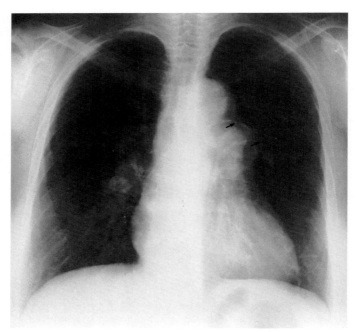

Figure 12.12. Patent ductus arteriosus with pulmonary hypertension and pulmonary calcification. This 53-year-old woman had calcification in her enlarged main pulmonary artery (*small arrows*). The pulmonary vessels also are pruned because of pulmonary hypertension, and a small amount of calcification is visible in the right pulmonary artery.

Like patients with tetralogy of Fallot, those with transposition of the great vessels or truncus arteriosus (Fig. 12.14) do not exhibit an enlarged main pulmonary artery segment. Rather, they exhibit an indistinguishable one. In both of these cyanotic diseases, pulmonary blood flow generally is increased if the patient lives to adulthood. The cardiac silhouette is globally enlarged, and the patient may have a right aortic arch. In those with truncus arteriosus, the pulmonary artery usually arises directly from the aorta, and varying degrees of pulmonary stenosis protect the lungs from being flooded with blood (because the pulmonary arteries are experiencing systemic pressures). The designations of type-1, -2, and -3 truncus arteriosus indicate the origin of the pulmonary artery, from a low level in the ascending aorta (i.e., type 1) to a progressively higher level in the ascending aorta (i.e., type 2 and 3). Type-4 truncus arteriosus actually is tetralogy of Fallot with pulmonary atresia (i.e., pseudotruncus), and in these patients, the pulmonary arteries arise from the descending aorta as bronchial arteries, which immediately anastomose with the pulmonary arteries in the lungs (Fig. 12.14*B*). Patients usually have increased blood flow to the lungs.

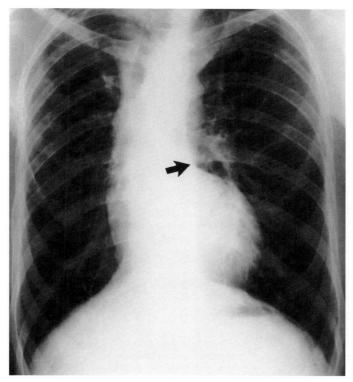

Figure 12.13. Boot-shaped heart secondary to tetralogy of Fallot. The cardiac apex is turned upward, and no main pulmonary artery segment can be seen (*arrow*). These two factors create the boot shape. Asymmetry of the pulmonary vessels also is seen because of a previous Blaylock procedure on the left and atresia of the right pulmonary artery.

In patients with transposition of the great vessels, a shunt must be present at the atrial or the ventricular level, or as a persistent PDA, to get blood to the lungs. The size of the shunt determines the amount of blood flow to the lungs. In adults, this blood flow usually is increased. Patients most likely to go undetected into adulthood are those with a common atrium or a common ventricle.

The two remaining right-to-left shunts both exhibit enlargement of the main pulmonary artery; thus, they can be differentiated from the other three cyanotic heart lesions. In tricuspid atresia (Fig. 12.2), an atrial shunt is necessary for the patient to survive, and a shunt at the ventricular or the ductus level is necessary to get blood to the lungs. Thus, these patients have multiple shunts. Patients who survive into adulthood usually have increased flow in their pulmonary vessels. The heart is globally enlarged as well, with enlargement of the main pulmonary artery segment and multiple chambers.

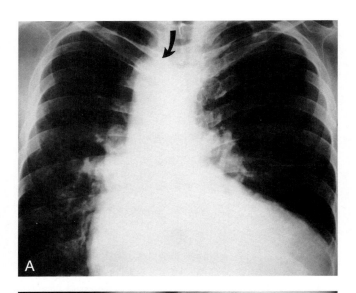

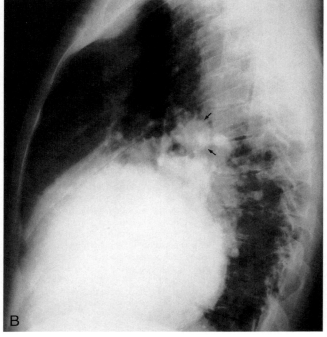

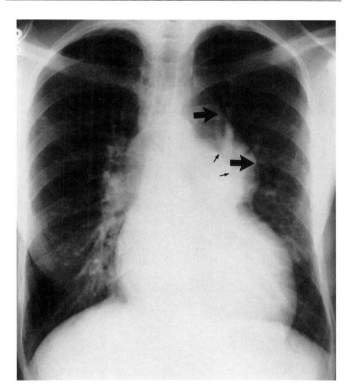

Figure 12.15. Total anomalous pulmonary venous return. The heart is enlarged, as is the main pulmonary artery segment (small arteries). The right superior vena cava and persistent left superior vena cava (*large arrows*) create the snowman appearance of the heart in this patient.

In total anomalous pulmonary venous return (TAPVR), the anomalous return can occur below the diaphragm (i.e., infracardiac) into the inferior vena cava, portal vein, hepatic vein, or other subdiaphragmatic vessels. In cardiac-type TAPVR, the anomalous return occurs at the cardiac level; this is the most unusual type of TAPVR.

In the third type of TAPVR (i.e., supracardiac), the shunt of the pulmonary veins to the right atrium occurs by the usual right superior vena cava and a per-

---

Figure 12.14. Truncus arteriosus. **A.** Posteroanterior film. The heart is hugely dilated, with no dilatation of the main pulmonary artery segment. A right aortic arch (*arrow*) is present as well. **B.** Lateral film. A vessel is seen posterior to the trachea (arrows) that represents bronchial vessels arising from the descending aorta. This is pathognomonic of a type-4 truncus arteriosus (i.e., pseudotruncus).

171

sistent left superior vena cava, thereby creating a heart that resembles a snowman (Fig. 12.15). These patients usually have a prominent main pulmonary artery segment, increased blood flow, and a globally enlarged heart. As with the adult transposition, those patients likely to survive into adulthood are those with a common atrium or common ventricle.

SUGGESTED READINGS

Elliott P, Schiebler GM. The x-ray diagnosis of congenital heart disease in infants, children, and adults. Springfield: Charles C. Thomas, 1968.

Spinola-Franco H, Fish BG. Radiology of the heart. New York: Springer-Verlag, 1985.

Index

Page numbers in *italics* denote figures; those followed by a t denote tables.

Index

Index

Index

Index

Fluid overload, pulmonary edema in, 6

Focal alveolar infiltrates (*see* Alveolar infiltrates, focal)

Focal asymmetry, and pulmonary abnormalities, 154–155

Focal interstitial lung disease (*see* Interstitial lung disease, focal)

Foreign body(ies), resorption atelectasis and, *66,* 67

Fracture healing, and rib lesions, 123

Fungal infection (*see also specific microorganism*)
  in focal alveolar infiltrates, 43–46
  in mediastinal mass, 137
  pleural effusion in, 108
  pulmonary nodules in, 85–87

G

Ganglioneuroma
  as extrapleural mass, 124–125
  as mediastinal mass, 144

Germ cell tumor, as mediastinal mass, 130

Ghon lesion, 41

Goiter, as mediastinal mass, 126–127, *128*

Goodpasture's syndrome, pulmonary hemorrhage in, 7

Granuloma (*see also* Wegener's granulomatosis)
  eosinophilic
    nodular interstitial pattern in, 28
    reticular interstitial pattern in, 22
  plasma cell, resorption atelectasis in, 67
  pulmonary nodules and, 73–74, *74*

H

Hamartoma(s)
  endobronchial, 67
  multiple pulmonary nodules and, 84
  solitary pulmonary nodules and, 71, *72*

Hamman-Rich syndrome, 18

Hampton's hump, 47

Heart (*see also* Cardiac *entries*)
  acquired disease of, 162–163
    pericardial effusion in, 162, *162*
    pulmonary hypertension in, *153,* 162–163

Heart (*continued*)
  anatomy of, 159–161, *160*
  congenital disease of, 163–172
    left-to-right shunts in, 164–166
    right-to-left shunts in, 166–172
    valvular lesions in, 163–164, *164*
  valvular disease of, *161,* 163

Heart failure, congestive, *157*
  alveolar edema secondary to, *159*
  pleural effusion in, 108
  subpulmonic effusion in, *103*

Heartworm, dog, 75

Hematopoiesis, extramedullary, as mediastinal mass, *147,* 148

Hemosiderosis, idiopathic, pulmonary hemorrhage in, 8

Hiatal hernia, 118, *118–119,* 120
  as mediastinal mass, 143–144

Histoplasma capsulatum
  in focal alveolar infiltrates, 45

Histoplasmosis
  and mediastinal masses, 137
  multiple pulmonary nodules in, 85, *85–86*

Hodgkin's lymphoma, as mediastinal mass, 135, *135*

Hounsfield units (HU), 73–74

Humidifier lung, 26

Hydatid disease, pulmonary nodules in, 89

Hyperlucency, of the lung, 92–93
  cause(s) of, 92–100
    asthma as, 95
    bullae as, 96
    chronic obstructive pulmonary disease as, 92–95
    congenital problems as, 95–96
    emphysema as, 92–95
    idiopathic bullous disease as, 97–98
  diffuse, 92–95
  focal, 95–100

Hypersensitivity lung
  chronic alveolar disease in, 12
  nodular interstitial pattern in, 26–27, *27*

Hypogammaglobulinemia
  bronchiectasis in, 33, *34*
  thymomas in, 128

I

Idiopathic bullous disease, 97–98, *98*

Idiopathic hemosiderosis, pulmonary hemorrhage in, 8

Index

Index

Index

Index

Index

Index

Index